Andreas Jel

Healthy with Tachyon

A Complete Handbook
Including Basic Principles and Application of
Products for Health and Wellness

Translated
by Christine M. Grimm

LOTUS PRESS
SHANGRI-LA

The information introduced in this book have been carefully re-searched and passed on to the best of my knowledge and conscious-ness. Despite this fact, neither the author nor the publisher assume any type of liability for presumed or actual damages of any kind that might result from the direct or indirect application or use of the statements in this book. The information in this book is intended for interested readers and educational purposes.

1st English edition 2000
© by Lotus Press
Box 325, Twin Lakes, WI 53181
The Shangri-La Series is published in cooperation
with Schneeloewe Verlagsberatung, Federal Republic of Germany
© 1999 reserved by Windpferd Verlagsgesellschaft mbH, Aitrang, Germany
All rights reserved
Translated by Christine M. Grimm
Cover illustration by Peter Ehrhardt
Interior illustrations and graphs by Peter Ehrhardt,
except on page 11 by David Wagner
Overall production: Schneeloewe, 87648 Aitrang, Germany

ISBN 0-914955-58-6
Library of Congress Catalog Number 99-97284

Printed in the USA

Table of Contents

Dedicated to my three children
Katharina, Sirius, and Jona
And to all living souls
Who teach me
In these times to plant trees
Whose fruits will nourish and delight them

Preface

The ideas and aids described by this book are integrated in the global vision of humanity at peace and in harmony with itself, attuned to nature and everything that exists. However, the starting point for realizing this vision and the key to overcoming the global crisis (which is the greatest challenge that we carry with us into the new millennium) is the individual human being—you and me.

Every crisis already has the seed for its solution existing within it! Once this seed has been found, we can cultivate it. The crisis can then quickly turn into a stepping stone to a higher level of order. It reveals itself to be the driving force, evolution, and therefore makes life possible in the first place.

Do you agree with me up to now? Are you aware that the solution to your own personal health and/or interpersonal crisis is important for the development of all human beings? Are you willing to turn the realization of the vision described above into a present for yourself and the world? If your answer is YES, then read this book very attentively! If your answer is NO, then perhaps you will find some evidence here that will allow you to consider such a YES.

I consider tachyonized tools, the topic of this book, to be essential aids in mastering crises on all levels of our being. They transform chaos (= entropy: term used in physics for constant decay of order) into harmony (= neg-entropy: development into increasingly more complex, higher order); they reverse the aging process and contribute to rejuvenation. In the first chapter of this book, I develop a model to illustrate this statement in an understandable way. This extensive image of the universe does justice not only to a spiritual view of the world that has developed over the course of the millennia but also includes the most highly developed insights and theories from modern physics and other sciences. It represents the reunification of spirituality and science. Consequently, it provides a well-founded and welcome insight into how tachyonized materials work, as well as insight into the game of life itself. If you are interested in a deeper understanding of the theoretic background and practical evidence, I invite you to study the book by David Wagner (the inventor of tachyonization) and Dr. Gabriel Cousens: *Tachyon*

Energy—A New Paradigm in Holistic Healing (published by North Atlantic Books 1999).

The second chapter, which discusses the various tachyonized products available at this time, encourages you to experiment on your own. The description of the individual materials and their possible areas of use, the stories and experiences of people who have used them, as well as background information on our bodies as the works of wonder that they are, will show how you can comprehend and support the process of healing and development. Then you can write your own stories about tachyon!

The third chapter goes into greater detail about our system's balancing responses to the use of tachyonized tools. Most of the concepts and measuring procedures that now serve us in crisis situations no longer function with non-frequency tachyons. Light is also shed upon this important experience. Ultimately, this is also an attempt to clarify the confusion caused by "imitations" and "further developments of the tachyon technology," which have appeared in the wake of the quick widespread acceptance and huge success of the genuine tachyonized materials.

Some possibilities of use for our everyday lives, as well as a selection of questions that are frequently asked on the topic of tachyon at seminars are included in the fourth chapter. This practice-oriented workbook and reader is rounded off by an insight into the global correlations and constantly growing number of possibilities for playing with tachyon.

I wish you much joy in reading this book and radiant health with tachyon.

Iserlohn, October 1999
Andreas Jell

Chapter 1

Theoretical Background

The Physics of Tachyons or: How our Universe Functions

Follow me into a fascinating world. Let's look over the shoulders of the brightest thinkers of the 20th century. We can watch quantum physicists wrest the secrets of Existence, unhinge the prevailing materialistic-mechanistic world view, and once again allow life its mystic nature, which is rooted in wonderment. The laws found in highly complex mathematical calculations and equally complicated scientific test series have their correlation in the spiritual and mystical experiences of all ages and cultures. The era of separating science and spirituality, which has led humanity into global chaos, has now come to an end. At the lowest point of this development and in the nick of time, we finally have the means to transform this chaos to a higher order. The direct use of tachyon energy through Tachyonized materials makes this possible, both on the individual level and the planetary level.

So what is tachyon? In terms of healing remedies and therapies, why is this tachyon energy so totally different from everything that has previously existed on the planet? How can we explain the tremendous success resulting from the use of Tachyonized tools? What does established science say about the place of tachyons in our universe?

The following model will provide the background for answers to these questions. It will also make it possible for us to achieve a more profound understanding of how our universe functions.

The Energetic Continuum

All forms in our world have vibrations. In the process, the FREQUENCY determines the character, the individual qualities of the vibration. It creates the difference between colors and sounds, as well as between brain cells and liver cells, between the rose and the bird and all the rest of the participants in this universe. Even the

9

hardest material, such as a diamond, is nothing other than the dance of vibrations at a specific frequency and in a particular form. The one thing that all forms of our universe have in common is that they move at less than the speed of light, which is the boundary within which our Creation takes place.

Quantum physicists see ZERO-POINT ENERGY as the beginning of this creation of all forms and frequencies. This ZPE has no form. It moves more quickly than light. It is present everywhere and at the same time (eternal) in the entire cosmos. It has no boundaries (infinite and inexhaustible) and contains within itself the total potential for a perfect development of our universe of forms. Various spiritual traditions also give their own names to this "energy." However, they warn that no name could ever completely embrace the "nameless." According to our physically oriented model, this means that no thought (= frequency = slower than light = limited in time and space) can understand the ZPE (= source of all frequencies = quicker than light = infinite and eternal). Please note that terms like prana, chi, orgone, od, etc. cannot be equated with zero-point energy since, without exception, these are energies that have already been manifested within a specific frequency range.

If the existence of ZPE had not been conclusively suggested by higher mathematics and the corresponding physical experiment series, no respectable physicist would have been willing to shatter the boundaries of recognized logic. This would have been comparable to exposing oneself in front of unenlightened colleagues with topics that have a suspicious religious quality to them. On the other hand, we find many different reports on how it is possible to experience the ZPE. Spiritual traditions possess a considerable repertoire to prepare the seeker for such an experience of unity with All That Is. But let's go back to physics!

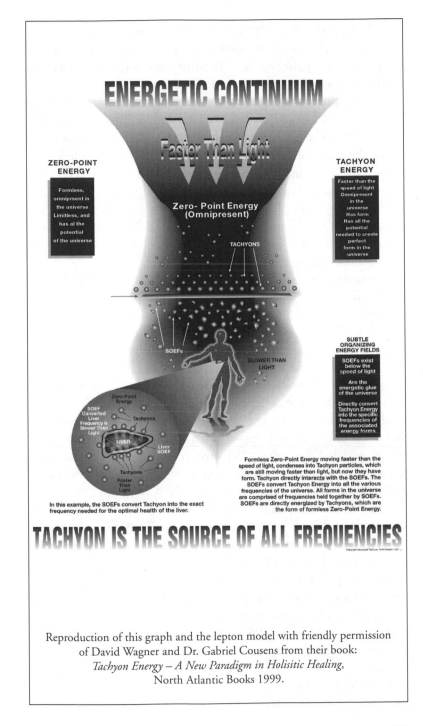

Reproduction of this graph and the lepton model with friendly permission
of David Wagner and Dr. Gabriel Cousens from their book:
Tachyon Energy – A New Paradigm in Holisitic Healing,
North Atlantic Books 1999.

The ENERGETIC CONTINUUM, as depicted on page 11, is a model. Similar to a map, it shows the path of a potential form to the point of its manifestation. The first step of this journey is the condensation of zero-point energy (ZPE) into TACHYONS. Tachyons are therefore ZPE that has been "condensed" into particle form. As such, in addition to the qualities of ZPE, their particle form also makes it possible for them to interact in the world of forms below the speed of light. Whenever this occurs, the result for the form world is balance and development into a higher order. The scientists speak of negative entropy, which means the reversal of decay and aging, the ordering of chaos, the transformation of inharmonious vibrations into harmonious ones. Before we take a more precise look at this contact and its effects, here is a further image to facilitate the understanding of zero-point energy:

Imagine that you are standing on the beach of a small island in the Pacific. An endless expanse of ocean extends as far as your eye can see. Now stretch out your hand to touch the entire ocean ... it doesn't work! This is what happens to everyone who tries to grasp the zero-point energy, whether with the hand, the mind, or any other technical (specific to one frequency) device. How could something infinite fit into the limited form of our hands? Now imagine that the pearly sea spray is dancing in the waves, splashing thousands of sparkling drops onto the cliffs. You stretch out your hand and catch one of these drops—a microcosm in drop form, with all the potential of the ocean. The drop (tachyon) allows us to grasp the infinite (zero-point energy) before it falls back into the ocean and becomes one with the whole again.

Now that we've had this little vacation in the Pacific, let's continue with quantum physics! In his book *The Physics of Tachyons*, Ernst L. Wall describes the elemental particle family of leptons. The smallest particle of this family is the PION. This tiny particle is kept in its position in a field (orbit) that vibrates just below the speed of light—therefore almost reaching this speed limit. The tachyon moves above this boundary at faster than the speed of light. If the action-ready orbit of the PION meets a TACHYON, a developmental process takes place that leads to a MUON, the next largest participant of the lepton family. The MUON has an orbit seven times larger than that of a PION. If the MUON once again meets a tachyon, the MUON develops in a leap into an ELECTRON with an orbit 207 times larger than that of the MUON. This process provides the basic building blocks for the perfect manifestation of a form. This form may be a liver cell, a human being, an ant, or a galaxy. All forms take this path! It is always the contact, the "inspiration" of the tachyons, that, like fertilization, sets this developmental process into motion.

Physics of Tachyons

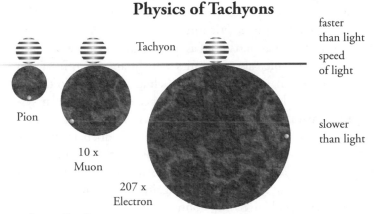

faster
than light
speed
of light

Tachyon

slower
than light

Pion

10 x
Muon

207 x
Electron

Lepton Family
By interacting with the tachyons, the SOEF of the respective leptons is capable of building, maintaining, and enacting a transformation process at an increasingly higher level of order (according to David Wagner).

The question as to what actually keeps the elemental particles in their order is not answered by Wall's research. We can find this answer in a model that the physician and scientist Dr. Gabriel Cousens first introduced during the 1980s: It places the effect of naturopathic therapies and, above all, the meaning of living nutrition into the light of the natural sciences. In his model of the SUBTLE ORGANIZING ENERGY FIELDS (SOEFs), he provided the theoretical background for numerous observations. One example of this model is that energy fields create the forms (frequencies). The opposite theory had previously been postulated—that the forms and the body are responsible for the energy fields. Here is a simple example of this idea: When we cut a tip off a living leaf and make a Kirlian photo of this leaf, we can continue to see a complete aura of the leaf, even at the place where the physical form has been cut. (Kirlian pictures are high-frequency photographs that allow a living being's subtle energy fields to become visible).

In Dr. Cousen's SOEF model, we can expand the model of the orbit as the field within which an object will probably stay to be actual energy forms. This reveals a further important step for scientifically understanding the creation process of this universe in its all-encompassing basic pattern: All forms/frequencies of this universe originate in a continuous process of condensation. This process is stimulated by tachyons and translated and controlled by SOEFs. Following this path, the perfect prototype is converted from the ZPE into its material and/or energetic form.

Everything that manifests itself as form in this universe has been shaped by a SOEF, which also continues to maintain this form. From the smallest currently known particles such as the pions, to the atoms, molecules, cells, organs, organisms, species, planets, solar systems, and galaxies...! SOEFs are what transforms the all-encompassing potential of the tachyons into the exact frequencies that are respectively required. This brings the above-mentioned units into the form intended by the source, as well as maintaining them and connecting them with this form. Once again: Everything that exists has an uninterrupted, dynamic connection with everything else through the SOEFs, as well as with the tachyon energy. As ZPE in particle form, the tachyon energy sustains the access to the infinite intelligence of the Creation. Here lies the biological key to Bell's theorem in which the physicist Bell, in a brilliant mathematical deduction, proclaimed the connection of all participants of this universe to be a physical reality.

Health and Disease in the Light of the New World View

For the first time in the history of the healing arts, the model of the energetic continuum and its scientific background allows a truly holistic look at the dynamics of disease and health. In our system of the energetic continuum, health is defined as the smooth, undisturbed condensation of the perfect blueprint down to its manifestation in physical form. This ideal blueprint, as laid out in the ZPE, finds its correlation in this world of forms. The parts of nature that have not been touched by "civilized" human beings reflect the wonderful, almost perfect interaction of all participating beings in fulfilling and developing the great musical score of life. Here diseases exist primarily in correlation with the preservation of a balanced development (for example, infectious diseases when there is over-population). Chronic illnesses like rheumatism, allergies, gout, dental cavities, diabetes, heart disease, etc., simply do not exist here. The SOEFs of the minerals, plants, animals, and the entire biosphere of our planet translate the potential of tachyon energy as extensively as possible into life forms. These life forms display a connected, balanced behavior toward members of the same species, as well as toward the entire biosphere.

In the language of the energetic continuum, disease means that during the condensation process, in the transformation of the blueprint from tachyons into the corresponding frequencies—something goes wrong. The perfect potential experiences a disturbed manifestation. In order to understand how something like this can occur, we must know that faster-than-light tachyon energy, and therefore all the perfect blueprints for frequencies and forms, exists everywhere in the universe and does so inexhaustibly; however, in order for them to be effective for us, they require access to our system, which exists at a speed slower than light.

Tachyon cannot go below the magical boundary of the speed of light in order to intervene actively in building the forms. This point is precisely what the quantum physicists have long speculated about. As we now know, tachyon needs the SOEFs for this purpose. Their condition determines the quality in which the universal blueprint can manifest itself. The paramount factor for influencing our SOEFs is FREE WILL, which makes it possible for us to stop or block the flow of the universal life energy (transference of tachyon into our individual energy system). Whenever we interrupt the condensation process (energy flow) from the more subtle areas of our EC, there will be an inadequate supply of ordering energy that maintains the natural functions in the subsequent, denser levels. This is how a blockage in the mental body (for example, the statement of the belief: "I am not desired") can block the harmonious flow of source energy and create stress. The next, denser emotional level forms the respective chaotic pattern (fear, spite, anger...) and passes on these disruptive patterns further into the physical body. Tensions and a variety of other disorders, such as stomach ulcers and digestive complaints, then may arise here. (See illustration on page 16)

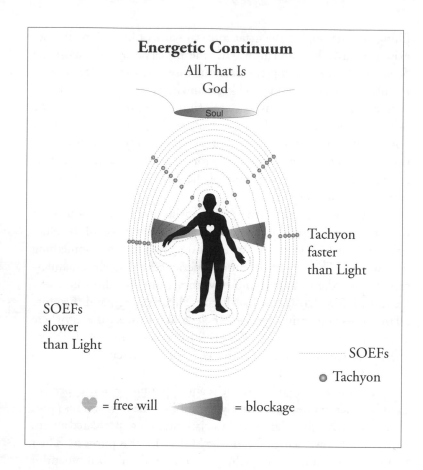

This sketch shows a longitudinal section through a human energy field. The dashed lines indicate SOEFs. Each of these SOEFs exists at the boundary of the speed of light. Tachyons enter from the space beyond the speed of light into interaction with individual SOEFs, in accordance with the charge of this field. The universal blueprint condenses step-by-step from the subtle areas at the outer edge, which also represent the higher frequency portions of our body, to the increasingly denser portions at the center of the picture. Blocked patterns are assumed from the respectively denser fields, which means a disturbed translation of the blueprint. This leaves its traces down into the physical levels of our being (disease, pain, malfunctions, etc.), indicated by the gray shadows behind the blockage.

Disorders in the physical body are always the ultimate and most highly condensed expression of a lacking contact between the corresponding SOEFs and the ordering energy of the tachyon. This leads to the SOEFs weakening. Consequently, this causes errors in the translation of the universal blueprint into our existence. At the end of this chapter, there is a practical example that uses the liver to depict this understanding of how diseases occur and what healing means.

But before we examine this aspect, let's take a look at the SOEFs: We already know that the SOEFs work just below the speed of light, obtaining the necessary energy from tachyons in order to build and maintain the optimal function of the frequencies and/or forms that correspond with them. Once the optimal balance of the form has been achieved, the SOEFs reduce their work until some sort of influence disrupts this balance, making a correction necessary. We experience this balancing act, which is concerned with developing the best possible form, as the dynamic alternation of order and chaos. In this sense, chaos plays the role of a teacher, providing the opportunity for learning to develop into increasingly higher levels of order. Disease makes it possible for us to correct a course that has deviated from our comprehensive plan in the Creation. It teaches us—and this particularly applies to pain—to precisely feel and perceive what elements have become imbalanced in our life.

Consequently, in this very elementary interplay of order, chaos, order, chaos, order, the task of the SOEFs is to keep the world of frequencies and forms in a feedback mechanism with itself. They also maintain its connection with the source (ZPE), via tachyon, and therefore enable an interactive evolution of all life.

The quality of this task directly depends upon the energetic state of the subtle field. Thanks to research findings by Dr. Gabriel Cousens (extensively documented in the book that he has written together with David Wagner: *Tachyon Energy, A New Paradigm in Holistic Healing*), we now know the following about the function of SOEFs:

According to the current state of knowledge, only two factors can build and strengthen the charge of human SOEFs: 1. Live food (rich in living, highly complex SOEFs) and 2. Tachyon energy.

If you expect the diverse healing methods to be listed at this point, you are mistaken. All systems of healing that have been developed on this planet up to now work on the basis of frequencies—

and **frequencies cannot strengthen SOEFs**. You will find scientific proof for this statement in the above-mentioned book by David Wagner and Dr. Gabriel Cousens. This proof was furnished by a renowned special laboratory in the USA that, for the past 18 years, has dedicated itself to the research of human DNA and the best way to attain mastery over the disease of "aging."

On the other hand, the influences that weaken or can destroy our SOEFs are quite numerous. I would just like to list their frontrunners (also see the topic of DETOXIFICATION).

1. **Influences from the outside** (Weakening of SOEFs through deprivation of ordering energy and blocking on the physical level)
   Dead food that has been denatured through cooking, radiation, microwaves, etc., chemical medications, herbicides, pesticides, exhaust fumes; dirty water lacking in energy, electrosmog, and noise—the accomplishments of our technically-oriented civilization.

2. **Influences from within** (Weakening of SOEFs through blocks in the energy flow of the energetic continuum on the mental and emotional levels)
   Blocked emotions, stress, stagnant patterns of belief—the reverse side of our free will.

Basically, every (!) supplied frequency vibrating outside of the area attended to by SOEFs and organized on a lower level weakens or destroys them. This occurrence depends upon the type, intensity, and length of this influence. Consequently, it is elementally very important that every application of frequencies serve the intention of healing: the precise nature of the disorder (form and frequency area), the cause, what specific healing frequency should be applied (such as acupuncture points, homeopathic remedies, phytogenic remedies, conversational strategies, medications, etc.), which dosage should be used, and when the application should be stopped!

The fulfillment of these requirements for the responsible approach to frequencies turns a good healer into an artist. This process demands that as we apply the art of healing, we precisely observe the effects of this influence on the patient. We must be capable of determining whether we are open to perceiving the indications that differentiate between a healing process and a worsening of these manifestations on all levels. It is also important to interpret them properly. Since a frequency (healing method) possesses no intelligence of its own to stop at the proper moment before the body has the possibility of ignoring the applied frequency, all the responsibility for this is in the hands of the people who use it. If, for example, we do not stop the application at the right point in time, we damage the SOEFs exactly as much as if we had made a mistake about the necessary intensity or in the choice of the right remedy.

Reputable therapists and those who work in the healing arts with a naturopathic orientation agree that these therapeutic possibilities are only meant to support the patients in activating their own powers of self-healing. "Nature heals"—this is obvious to anyone working in the healing arts who has shed the healer ego and approaches the unbelievable complexity of the system "human being and disease" with humility. In terms of our model, this means that only intact, freely vibrating, and connected SOEFs heal! In holistic healing, frequencies and healing remedies serve solely as crutches or blockage-dissolvers on the level of disturbed form. Only when the body has rebuilt the corresponding SOEFs and these once again assume their intended function does healing occur. Then the crutches that have been used must be put aside immediately. Otherwise, they would once again destroy the balance created by the SOEFs.

Up until the invention of Tachyonization, it was only possible to support the powers of self-healing by supplying highly charged, living SOEFs. One possibility of this is from raw fruit and vegetables that have been naturally cultivated. Live food is just as essential for healing and development as avoiding the SOEF-damaging influences mentioned above. Under the descriptions of the Tachyonized tools in the next chapter, there are explanations of how you can simply and effectively protect yourself against disruptive influences in many cases.

Tachyon Energy—Totally Different

With all the preceding background knowledge, the focus of the unique effect in the use of tachyons for healing and development becomes clear: When tachyon energy is supplied by means of the Tachyonized tools presented in this book, **the disturbed SOEFs are strengthened**. According to their very individual possibilities and dynamics, the SOEFs recreate the optimal balance for the forms that they have shaped and continue to maintain them. Accordingly, tachyon energy is the most direct way of strengthening the SOEFs' powers of self-healing. In contrast to the use of frequencies, there can be *no overdose* of tachyon: *no application is too long*, and we don't need to be concerned about using the right remedy since all Tachyonized tools only give off tachyon energy. This energy contains *all the potential for everything in the universe* and for *all forms* in an optimal manner. This also means, for example, that the same Tachyonized glass cell can be used on the head, abdomen, arm, or anywhere else. On the basis of this abundance of tachyon energy, the SOEFs transform precisely the frequencies that enable an optimal functioning of the corresponding form (organ, gland, chakra, injured body part, etc.). Once the balance (healing) has been attained, the SOEF ends this process on its own. A continued supply of tachyon energy has no further effect.

Without exception(!), all manifestations and symptoms in correlation with the use of Tachyonized materials are the regulating, balance-creating action of the SOEFs! We call the results of this cleansing process *detoxification*! Whenever a person using tachyon experiences detoxification, it should be welcomed as the necessary clean-up action. If this process takes place too vehemently, it usually suffices to reduce the amount of tachyon energy supplied, allowing the corresponding SOEFs to complete their work in a slower and gentler way. It is also possible to find a specially trained tachyon practitioner who has the remedies and knowledge to help a person through such detoxification processes with great speed and grace (see TLC Bars and Bifurcation).

The Model of the Energetic Continuum in the Practice

Here is a summary of how the model of the SOEFs and the energetic continuum (EC) are translated into the practice. All frequencies and forms of this universe, from the smallest pion to the largest galaxy, are shaped and kept in their individual form by corresponding SOEFs. Through contact with these tachyons, these SOEFs create the exact frequencies necessary for manifesting the perfect blueprint from the ZPE in our universe of time and space.

In the depiction of the EC on page 11, the human liver is used as an example. All information and frequencies that the liver requires as a whole for its optimal functioning are controlled through the corresponding SOEF. Integrated in the superordinate body SOEFs, it coordinates the interplay of all the cells, tissue, molecules (including metabolism), atoms, and elemental particles that form the liver, down to the pion. This liver SOEF translates all the information for the function and structure from the perfect, individual blueprint imparted by the tachyons. It builds the physical form of the liver, including its many levels of tasks, from the components of the supplied nutrition. The more highly organized the SOEFs of this food are, for example, organically grown, raw fruit and vegetables, the better the building blocks will be that our liver has available to it to fulfill its tasks. If we subject ourselves to liver-weakening frequencies like alcohol, medication, meat, certain drugs, and poisoning through disturbed intestines, we hinder the transformation of tachyon energy into a balanced liver functioning. We achieve the same through our ability to create blockages in the energetic continuum through our FREE WILL.

In the case of the liver, for example, our alternative of constantly suppressing our anger blocks the liver SOEF to the extent that metabolic performance on the physical level can no longer be adequately coordinated. Once the critical point at which the liver SOEF no longer can adequately perform its supportive function is attained, the liver deteriorates into a lower level of the order (also see the topic *Bifurcation* in the section on the TLC Bars). We call this disease (for example: fatty liver, cirrhosis, and cancer).

Since a healthy liver resonates in a specific, relatively constant frequency range, it is possible to stop the deterioration of the form into chaos by supplying the corresponding frequencies (healing remedies), provided that the right remedy is applied at the right intensity. However, without simultaneously strengthening the SOEFs, no healing takes place. Putting aside the crutches leads to further deterioration.

Depending on the condition of the entire body's SOEFs, the damaged SOEFs of the liver can be restored again when the corresponding building materials are supplied through live food and the harmful influences are stopped and/or cleaned out. This means that if frequency remedies are used for too long, or false frequencies and strategies are applied, the deterioration is intensified because the body possesses no feedback mechanism against outside frequencies. Heal-

Fundamentals of Tachyon Energy

ZERO-POINT ENERGY (ZPE)	TACHYONS
Faster than the speed of light	Faster than the speed of light
Formless	Limitless
Limitless	Everywhere at the same time
Everywhere at the same time	No frequency
No frequency	No spin
No spin	No gravitation
No gravitation	Source of all energies
Source of all energies	100% perfect potential
100% perfect potential	of the entire universe
of the entire universe	within itself
within itself	ZPE condensed into form

SOEFs
(Subtle Organizing Energy Fields)

Exist just below the speed of light
Translate blueprints from the tachyons into the corresponding frequency to maintain the energy forms that are integrated into them.
Are intensified by tachyons,
Weakened by outside frequencies, especially those that are dissonant and chaotic
Create, maintain, and develop all forms that exist.
Divine feedback mechanism.

FREQUENCIES
Created and kept in form by SOEFs
Have vibration and/or spin
Move more slowly than the speed of light
Have a form
Interaction only with other frequencies, for example: through resonance, modulation, interference
Possess no intelligence

ing the liver with the help of frequency-specific methods requires an inseparable interplay of the following functions: support provided by the exact healing remedies through qualified healing practitioners and, to an even greater extent, a conscious change of lifestyle from one that creates illness into one that promotes life.

Even Hippocrates, according to whose example all physicians must swear their oath, recognized the limitations of his healing arts in exactly this point. The following was supposedly written on the entrance door to his practice: *"Sufferer, as long as you are not willing to ban the cause of your suffering from your life, go away from my doorstep so that you do not steal my precious time!"* The essential aspect for every healing and development, namely to learn from the suffering and develop into increasingly higher orders, ultimately also decides whether the use of tachyon energy leads to the desired result.

The incomparable effect of using tachyon energy lies in the activation of the SOEFs. This cannot be achieved by any manner of influencing the frequency! When both sufferers and professional healing practitioners use Tachyonized remedies, none of the risks and side effects that are characteristic of frequency-specific therapy methods occur. Applications with Tachyonized tools (which will be introduced in the next section), for example, only strengthen the respectively affected SOEFs for our affected liver or for all the other disorders that we develop. For their part, these SOEFs then introduce and monitor the healing process until the perfect balance—the natural function—has been restored. Once this state is achieved, an increased supply of tachyons no longer has an effect. The absorption of live food and the avoidance of harmful influences also play, as already mentioned, a decisive role in the application of tachyon energy. Personal growth as a result of our disorders and learning from the consequences of our FREE WILL still always remain the primary condition for true healing and development.

Congratulations! You have succeeded in feeling your way through a highly topical theory that is unavoidable for an understanding of the tachyon effect. At this point, I will leave it up to you to draw your own conclusions about what the possibility of directly using tachyons through Tachyonized materials means for humanity. Humanity is not only in the process of discharging and exhausting the SOEFs of its individuals, but also those of the entire biosphere. Consider what it means to you as an individual to have an aid available that makes it possible to get off this treadmill. You can make a considerable contribution to the healing of the entire planet with your own personal healing.

The model presented here provides us with the fundamentals to answer the most frequent questions that arise during the application of Tachyonized products. With this knowledge in our hands, we no longer need to relegate healing that takes place with tachyon energy to the realm of miracles. We recognize the naturalness of these processes and know how we can support them. If you want them to, they are willing to create your individual plan with the help of the next chapter. This will show you how you can use these wonderful tachyon tools to support your own healing and development, as well as that of your family, patients/clients, friends, pets and other animals, plants, and the entire planet.

Before we completely immerse ourselves in the practical aspects of tachyon technology, it is important for you to learn a bit more about the background of this invention. So follow me through time and space into the life of a man with extraordinary gifts:

David Wagner and the Process of Tachyonization

David Wagner's career as a technician and inventor already began when he was 10 years old. With the invention of a generator that caused three light bulbs to glow, he won the first prize in a contest. During this time, everyone in his circle of relatives and acquaintances feared him because of his insatiable curiosity. This curiosity was aimed at the content and function of all the electrical household devices, which he naturally also had to take apart for the benefit of his urge for knowledge. Once this thirst for knowledge was quenched and the magic revealed, frequently just the disassembled remains were left.

His ability to see energy flowing, in both living beings and technical devices, made it possible for him to have a deep understanding of how life functions on the various levels of manifestation. Before a serious accident made him a total invalid, he was the leading engineer at one of the largest American electronics firms. In this function, he coordinated the work of 134 employees developing hardware and software for the surface-to-air monitoring of all American airports. In addition to this task, it was possible for him to do research in his technical laboratory, equipped state-of-the-art devices covering about 400 square meters. This research followed in the steps of Nikola Tesla and his discoveries in the area of free energy.

Parallel to his work with technology and science, David Wagner's life has been characterized by spirituality and the healing arts. At the age of 7 years, a completely new experience of this world suddenly opened up to him. In a flash, his accustomed world of solid forms transformed into an uninterrupted flowing of energy. This occurrence additionally confronted him with the ability to "hear" other people's thoughts so that he initially couldn't differentiate them from spoken words. Among other things, at school this led to situations that often ended with a beating from an angry teacher who had received answers to his thoughts, which were completely different from his spoken words. On the whole, learning to live a normal life with this newly acquired ability was a difficult process for little David. So he naturally didn't succeed in fitting in completely with social standards.

At the time when he became a leading technician at the above-mentioned company, he had a regular job with a very good salary, was married, had a son, but also led meditation groups and ran a store with crystals from his own mines. These mines had already belonged to his family for three generations, and he used these crystals when holding workshops on healing and the laying-on of hands.

The process of unifying both aspects of his life was first initiated when a serious accident tore him out of this course of his life, with which he had been highly satisfied. Proclaimed in his morning meditation as a day that would change his life for the better, it ended for David Wagner with a triple prolapsed disk. While moving from one office to another, a full filing cabinet fell on him and suddenly ended his career as a technician, group leader, and happy husband and father. He was diagnosed as incurable after a number of painful and unsuccessful operations. Now David Wagner was unable to walk, stand, sit, or lay down without pain. Classified as a total invalid for the rest of his life, it appeared that everything had now come to an end.

At the deepest point of his crisis, after bouts of anger and doubts about his fate, he remembered the way in which he previously had obtained answers to his burning questions. Instead of complaining and cursing, he now asked the simple question that had never occurred to him during the entire time of his suffering: "What is the next step for my healing? What can I do?" At this moment, all of his technical and spiritual experiences and discoveries formed an image that climaxed in the blueprint and understanding of exactly how Tachyonization functions. (At this point, I would like to point out that many world-changing inventions and perceptions were born in this, or a similar, manner: for example, Albert Einstein's theory of relativity, Niels Bohr's atom model, Kekule's benzol structure...).

However, in order to put his blueprint into action, some obstacles still had to be overcome. By using medication, he got the pain under control. With the advance payment of his own and his brother's inheritance—and everyone thinking that he was totally crazy – David Wagner succeeded in having the necessary components for his Tachyonization chamber built. This wasn't (and still isn't) an easy thing to do since these components have no meaningful task in any type of technology currently existing on the planet. The company in question that was capable of building something like this was naturally aware of the situation. Only with the necessary "small change" was it possible to talk the person who ran it into manufacturing such "nonsense."

When it was time to launch this first device, David Wagner sent his family out of the house, programmed the emergency number into the telephone, and started up the machine from an adjacent room using a remote control—you never know exactly what could happen! During the six hours in which the prototype of the Tachyonization chamber ran smoothly, it was possible for David Wagner to recognize all the flaws of its construction. When the machine went up in flames after this time, it was already clear how it would be possible for the next device to run for 14 days. David Wagner knew that at least these 14 days would be necessary in order to change the subatomic structure of the material in the chamber so that it could itself become a permanent antenna for the tachyon energy.

And this is how things worked out. The first Tachyonized material, glass cells, served to completely reinstate the health of his back within six months, meaning unrestricted flexibility with complete freedom from pain. David Wagner had achieved his goal and the invention of this Tachyonization process had fulfilled its purpose.

Since it was only natural for his private life to expand into the outside world again, friends and acquaintances wanted to know how he had experienced such healing. After the one or the other application for friends, the demand quickly exploded and his office transformed itself into a small clinic. When two orthopedic doctors who operated a pain clinic in the same city ultimately experienced the fantastic effect of tachyons on themselves, the whole business got completely out of hand. Additional chambers had to be built because clients and patients wanted to take the Tachyonized materials with them. A clinic was opened, the only one working with tachyons, to find out what this invention was actually capable of. Here and in what was soon to be 20 additional practices, people researched, experimented, and compiled the experiences with thousands of individuals before the first Tachyonized article was released to the public. This took place in 1990.

Arising from the motivation of healing himself, which David Wagner had not succeeded in doing with any of the healing methods known at that time, the tachyon technology developed explosively. The potential of this technology includes the healing and spiritual development of all human beings who focus their free will onto it and are open to it. As a further consequence, the possibilities of using Tachyonized tools also include the healing and balancing of our biosphere, which has become increasingly imbalanced through the merciless application of destructive technologies.

David Wagner comprehended this potential and recognized that the foremost opportunity for showing a way out of the worldwide crisis is the development of human consciousness. In this sense, he also understood his invention of Tachyonization to be an aid for each individual human being to once again find the connection to his or her own divinity. From this very direct process of reconnection, we can follow our individual path of healing and development, integrated in the evolution of the entire family of humanity and the biosphere of this wonderful blue jewel, Earth.

The Technology of Tachyon

It would be possible to patent the process of Tachyonization 100%. However, David Wagner decided to not disclose the secret (yet). In contrast to many of his predecessors who have researched free energy, his invention will not be lost should David Wagner change his form of existence. His videos, blueprints, and all the necessary information has been distributed to various places and is ready for someone else to immediately continue his work. An attempt on his life in 1992 made David Wagner sensitive to this topic. During the early phases of my contact with tachyons, I was so enthusiastic that I wanted the whole world to know about it. I thought each of us should Tachyonize, but this enthusiasm soon gave way to the sober perception that this new technology, like every tool, could not just be used for the benefit of all people. And so I am very glad that the Existence has chosen someone whose intelligence and integrity have not been shattered by economic motives to manage this gift. David Wagner's love of humanity and the Existence represent the sole criterion for his actions.

Consequently, I cannot explain how Tachyonization functions since no one except David Wagner knows. But I can reveal here how it does not function: The Tachyonization process does **not** work with frequencies, spin, manipulation, or transference. It is **not** a high-frequency coil technique. It does **not** use tones, is **not** a vacuum, and has **nothing** to do with radionic devices (such as the SE5) and transference of information. Tachyonization does **not** use any sacred geometry to inform products **nor** does it require meditation and prayer. It is **not** possible to inform tachyon energy in any way, nor is it negative or positive. It does **not** spin to the right or left. It is **not** strong, weak, or neutral. The process is not based on photon technology. It uses **neither** crystals **nor** orgone technology. It employs **no** magnets. Tachyon works completely **independent** of the respective user.

I have learned to live with these open questions. The countless experiences that I have had myself, with my family, friends, patients, and participants in groups, has made this much easier for me. Experiencing David "live" has shifted this uncertainty of not knowing exactly what is happening here completely into the background. For years, I have been involved in therapy and training groups, have sat at the feet of some of the masters, and have developed a sense for dreamers and realists, geniuses and swindlers, the selfless and the egonauts. I have learned to take a very precise look at things and recognize what functions and what does not. So now I can say from the bottom of my much-traveled heart: Tachyon works, David Wagner personally takes the path that he offers, and the driving power behind it is the most rewarding in the entire universe. So—what are we still waiting for?

Chapter 2

Tachyonized Products

Preliminary Remarks

This chapter on Tachyonized products is classified into various groups. The sole purpose of this is to provide a better survey of the products available at this time. The essential point and common denominator of the tools introduced here is their antenna effect for tachyon energy. In this sense, they all have the same effect! And so the very best tachyon tool is not to be found in a specific section but always the one that you have available. The specific needs, the way in which tachyon energy reaches or enters the body in the most meaningful or comfortable manner are all secondary. This is why various aids have been developed. These materials never emit the healing effect, they "just" transduce tachyon energy. But this doesn't heal either. Only the body's own SOEFs heal when they translate the potential of tachyons into the corresponding form/frequency. So the choice of the tool is determined by the simple application, the necessary intensity, and the way we can best approach the disrupted SOEFs.

The ideas and possibilities introduced in this book, and particularly in this chapter, are not meant to replace the necessary support of a qualified healthcare professional. In the case of any health disorder for which you cannot—or believe that you cannot—assume full responsibility for its healing, I advise that you seek the professional support of a qualified practitioner of the healing arts, as mentioned above.

Even if the results that have been achieved when employing Tachyonized tools around the world may suggest this, there can basically be no promise of healing. No one who can be taken seriously can make this type of promise. The FREE WILL of each individual still remains the key for healing, and tachyon energy in no way disregards or undermines it. The FREE WILL also determines how much we support the healing process, which is set into motion by the tachyons, through the appropriate lifestyle. Only when the FREE WILL is used together with tachyon energy do those unbelievable turns of fate occur that each of us would call miraculous healing if we were not familiar with the background presented here.

I have chosen the practical examples from my own surrounding world (family, practice, and friends). This means I know most of those involved personally and only my own perspective stands between the experiences that they have had and my notes. I also did not intentionally search out the "best." Instead, I cite the cases that spontaneously came to mind while writing. I am not interested in wanting to prove something—the experiences had by those who have used tachyon energy will encourage and inspire readers to have their own.

Important note!

Because of the great worldwide success with Tachyonized tools, there are unfortunately some people who have given their old, frequency-specific tools the new varnish of "tachyon" or "tachyonization." At this point, I would like to point out that the materials and experiences described in this book are solely connected with the Tachyonized products manufactured by David Wagner. For your safety, these are marked with the protected logo of Advanced Tachyon Technologies:

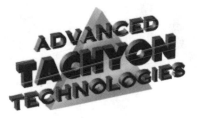

In order to avoid any errors, you should only purchase Tachyonized products from authorized distribution partners of ATT.

Products with a Focused-Directional Tachyon Field

The process of Tachyonization transforms hard materials into antennas that focus tachyon energy in just one direction. This results in an enormous effect for its use against pain and other disorders on the physical level.

As a reminder: the denser the tachyon field, the more quickly the SOEFs will become balanced. The size of the directional products determines the size of the region in which this regulation takes place. This results in the rule of thumb: **Cover the entire pain area as much as possible.**

Among the focused products are:

silica disks

glass cells

jewelry

Flexcell 100

Happy Soles.

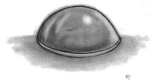

Tachyonized Silica Disks

Tachyonized silica disks offer a great variety of application possibilities. The basic material is silicon dioxide (quartz) in powder form, which is pressed into disks under high pressure. The high molecular density leads to a correspondingly dense (strong) tachyon field, with a length of approx. 5 meters in the diameter of the disk (approx. 10 cm).

Tip: The best way is to keep your Tachyonized silica disks in CD covers to protect them from breakage. However, if one should happen to break, this does not influence the Tachyonization. It only influences the direction in which the tachyons flow: the more powder, the more the fields are unfocused.

Application Possibilities:

Electrosmog: Correcting Negative Effects of Extra Low-Frequency Alternating-Current Fields (ELFs)

Background knowledge: Electrosmog

Long before David Wagner invented the process of Tachyonization, an important part of his work as a scientist was dedicated to the problem of mastering electrosmog with its catastrophic effects on human beings. We thank his research as the technical manager of the largest American electronics company at that time for the discovery of the disease-causing effects of the ELFs.

The harmful effect of electricity in residences primarily results from the chaotic frequency patterns that occur in the transformation of high-voltage current into household electricity—the superordinate SOEFs decay into a lower order. The result of this is that the form of a harmonious sinus wave cannot be maintained and is torn apart because of the alternation between the phases. If such a disturbed pattern meets an ordered frequency, equalization occurs. The chaos organizes itself at the cost of the higher order. For people, animals, and plants, this universal dynamic means the loss of organizing energy (vitality), and weakened and discharged SOEFs, as soon as they are subjected to these chaotic, "unraveled" EM fields.

Important: The ELF field as such is not the feared electrosmog, but the chaotic structure of this field that draws off coherent energy (vital force) in order to harmonize itself.

Tachyonized silica disks, attached with the tachyon field in the direction of the main fuse, already harmonize the chaotic vibrational structure of the alternating current in the fuse box. This consequently corrects the negative effects of all the connected electrical equipment. It puts an end to the discharging of live food such as fresh fruit and vegetables by the refrigerator, juicer, or mixer. Whether the hairdryer or the computer, including the monitor, the lamps or cables and wiring—the entire living area becomes free of electrosmog!

Various studies on lab mice have shown that mice forced to live behind a continually running computer monitor survived for no longer than three months; a comparison group, without the influence of the monitor, lived six months.

We additionally observed mice in the area of a monitor of the same brand as in the above test series, but our monitor had its negative effects corrected with a Tachyonized disk. The first mouse of the group died after twelve months! The rest of the test crew, which had grown into a sizable population, was set free.

Similar circumstances resulted from experiments with fruit-fly populations.

Intelligence and concentration tests on students subject to the influence of computer monitors with the negative effects corrected yielded performance increases of up to about 180 percent in comparison to a group without a monitor. The group behind the monitor that had not had its negative effects corrected experienced about a 60 percent decrease in performance.

These results are also the reason why Tachyonized silica disks are available in almost every Japanese computer store and one of the largest computer companies in Japan installs them as standard equipment in their monitors.

If it isn't possible for you to get to the fuses (for example, at work or in the office), you can correct the negative effects of the computer monitor by attaching a Tachyonized silica disk with the tachyon field (side with writing) toward the device.

Report on Experience
A course participant from Munich reported that her cat had stopped sleeping in her home from the moment that the silica disk was attached to the fuse box. (Cats tend to be attracted to places with

negative energy.) Up to that point, the cat had completely ignored all attempts to move it out of the living area. Now it slept in the heating cellar. Interestingly enough, the heating cellar was the only room in the house that hadn't had its negative effects corrected because a different electric circuit supplied it.

Water Quality

Living water plays an essential role for our health. The rapid deterioration of the drinking-water quality is being countered by numerous attempts to revitalize it. Under the topic of *Tachyonized Water*, you will find some fundamentals about the meaning of water quality for living beings. At this point, I would like to point out how simple and effective tachyons are when used for the improvement the water quality.

Charging water with the Tachyonized silica disk: Simply place the glass or bottle of water on the disk (side with writing facing upward!) The SOEFs of the water immediately begin to balance themselves and optimize the structure of the water molecules. Even after just a few minutes, the result is a distinct increase in the biological activity. Its maximum intensity is achieved after about 6 to 8 hours. This time period results from the mass inertia of the water molecule. Independent of the surrounding energy, the water once again discharges itself when it is taken from the disk. However, even after one week, the quality is still far above the initial value. Set onto the disk, many bottles and a good quantity of fruit and vegetables can be charged within the overall field, which is 5 meters long!

Sprouts grow in an optimal balance on Tachyonized silica disks, which usually also means more quickly and to larger size. A simple test of this will convince anyone.

Plants generally love living water. They thrive luxuriantly and have radiant health when they are regularly given charged water.

Wristband (around a glass), glass cells, Flexcells, or Happy Souls also can be used to charge water. If the entire amount of water is not located within the tachyon field, charging will simply take somewhat longer.

Report on Experience

Swimming-pool and therapy-pool owners who have attached the Tachyonized silica disks to their pools report a distinct increase in the feeling of well-being when people are in the water. Furthermore, it was clear that fewer measures were necessary to keep the pool clean. When disinfecting with substances containing chlorine, remember that chlorine returns more quickly to its gaseous original state in a tachyon field. The resulting increased water quality also allows a smaller concentration of such toxic substances.

When considering how many Tachyonized silica disks are required, the following applies: the more disks, the more quickly the maximum charge will be achieved. Then this level can be maintained with one single disk.

As a reminder: Water charged in the tachyon field is NOT Tachyonized. In order to Tachyonize water, it must go through David Wagner's Tachyonization process for 14 days. Only here can a subatomic restructuring occur, which will allow it to become an antenna for tachyon energy.

Sleep Quality

Background Knowledge: Sleep

When we sleep, we go through a number of phases in rhythmic alternation that accompany the corresponding brain activity (frequency patterns). The dream phases take place during the time near the waking state, while the greater portion and most important regeneration work of our physical body occurs in the relatively short periods in the dreamless, unconscious depths. During this time, we again fill up the emptied stores in order to be adequately equipped for the next day. An undisturbed deep sleep leads to a feeling of being fit and well-rested in the morning, no matter whether we have slept 5 or 10 hours: Not the length of the sleep but its depth plays a decisive role. In addition to other disruptive influences, above all it is intensive dream activity, usually provoked by blocked or stagnated energies in our emotional body, that prevent an immersion into these areas.

Here as well, we can meaningfully apply a Tachyonized silica disk: attached to the head of the bed, with the writing pointed in the direction of the feet, about 10 centimeters (4 inches) above or below the surface of the body. In no case should the tachyon field point through the body since this would trigger balancing processes that could prevent the person from sinking into the necessary depths of sleep. The goal is simply to have a continuous "stream" of vital energy flowing through the subtle areas of the energy field in order to harmonize stagnation and excess movements during sleep.

Many users have reported more intensive dream activities, mainly during the first nights after attaching the disk. But to their amazement, most of them felt like they had a good night's sleep and were fit the next morning.

The same support can also be easily and effectively implemented at the sickbed, especially for those who are seriously ill and dying. Here it is important to maintain the flow of vital energies, stimulate them whenever the recovery process needs to be supported, or when we want to make it easier for another person to change over into the next form of existence.

Had the following story not happened within my own family, I would not have considered it possible.

Report on Experience

A 60-year-old man was brought to the hospital with an acute kidney failure. The catastrophic lab values agreed with the overall picture: He could no longer be helped. For this reason, the physicians did not take any action except assigning him to a room in which he could spend the night—which he would not live through—without being disturbed. Despite this pessimism, his daughter hung a silica disk on his bed since "it can't hurt and maybe it will help!" The next morning, the night nurse came into the room and, instead of finding a corpse that had to be taken care of, she found a patient sitting up in bed and complaining. After one week, he left the clinic on foot and took along the disk. However, he didn't believe it was the source of his recovery.

Cleansing of Crystals

Because of their specific structure in connection with gravitational forces, crystals are capable of binding and intensifying electromagnetic vibrations, meaning chaotic, technical fields, as well as frequencies in the range of human thoughts and emotions. Washing crystals under running water is one method of cleaning them, but not very effective. "Cleansing" crystals in table salt can be harmful to them: When moist, table salt expands more than the quartz crystal and breaks fine tears into its surface. Not everyone who loves crystals knows the techniques of mentally cleansing them, which is the most effective process apart from tachyon energy. This means that many crystals stand around in homes and stores, continuously intensifying and transmitting the collected, chaotic vibrational patterns.

In a tachyon field, it isn't possible for dissonant, chaotic vibrations to cling to the crystals. So they can be quickly cleaned without too much trouble. They can also be freed from and protected against all outside energies. Milky clouding may turn transparent, sometimes even after just a few days on the silica disk.

Did you know that water is only a liquid starting at 60 degrees Celsius (140 degrees Fahrenheit)? Below this point it behaves like a liquid crystal. The exact interface of optimal formability and stability is found at 37 degrees Celsius (98.6 degrees Fahrenheit). As in the above-described crystals, dissonant outside energies can cling to the body water (liquid crystal) and make life difficult for us. However, with the help of tachyons we can effectively protect ourselves against this problem. In my healing work, I no longer feel exhausted or drained. I also no longer suffer from abysmal tiredness, even after intensive treatment days or on weekends, since I started using tachyons.

Application for Plants

Indoor plants are the most important connection to nature in our living space. They assume a decisive role in the creation of a live atmosphere. Everything that applies to the above statements about crystals and water naturally is also true of plants as well.

Watering with charged water on a regular basis, as well as the direct use of silica disks, can primarily help cut flowers, sick plants (with pest infestation), freshly repotted, and newly purchased plants to reintegrate themselves into a nature context. This leads to luxuriant growth and strong powers of resistance. As thanks for the tachyon application, plants that have been supported in this manner provide a wonderful room climate in which a human being can feel well.

Driving a Car

The lacking ground contact, together with electromagnetic isolation, can lead to a variety of impairments in a car. Becoming tired too quickly and disturbed concentration are part of everyday driving, particularly on longer stretches.

A silica disk attached to the inside of the roof in a CD cover, for example, with the tachyon field focused through the body (writing facing downward) balances dissonant patterns like stress and annoyance, tensions in the back, concentration disturbances. This can also prevent false judgments and wrong reactions. Breaks become more restful and even long trips in the car lose their energy-robbing effect.

Additional aids for drivers are: Sleep Pad, Life-Padd, Vitalizer II or Flexcell 100, silk meditation wrap, eye pillow or eye mask for breaks, Happy Souls, headband, wristbands, Ultra-Freeze (on the neck), and Tachyonized Klamath Lake Algae.

Tachyonized Glass Cells

Like all silicon compounds, glass is among the materials that respond particularly well to Tachyonization. The tachyon field of all glass cells is approx. 3 centimeters (1.2 inches) long. The size corresponds with the diameter of the respective cell. The balancing in the tachyon field relates to the entire organism. However, particularly for focused products, the main effect occurs precisely within the area of the directed field.

Example
My wife tripped over our dog one night, hitting her right upper arm on the edge of a dresser. The next morning, a gigantic, dark-blue bruise marked the entire upper arm. We stuck nine pieces of colored 24mm cells onto it. The next day, the skin beneath the cells had completely regained its normal color again—but the deep-violet hued skin in the area between the cells was raised like a silhouette.

Possibilities of Application
There are two types of Tachyonized cells: colored and colorless (clear or opal). The tachyon field is emitted from the flat side of all colored cells and the round side of the colorless cells.

The following sizes of colored and colorless cells are available: 13mm, 15mm, 24mm, and 30mm. The following special sizes are only available in the colorless cells (tachyon field flows from the round side).

The 8mm cells are meant for application on acupuncture points. To do this, it's best to lay the cell with the flat side on an adhesive fleece and apply light pressure with the round side on the skin.

Important: Even when used for a longer period of time, there can be no overcharging of the meridians since tachyon creates only the conditions for balance. Once this has been achieved, there are no more reactions on the part of the body, even if the cells continue to be worn.

13mm and 15mm for small joints, throat and neck, insect bites, warts, and other small-surface areas of application.

24mm and 30mm on muscular pain points (trigger points), anywhere they can be easily adhered to. The rule of thumb is: Always stick on the Tachyonized cells so that they cover the entire surface on the disturbed area (see blue bruise story above).

75mm glass cells are made for charging water, crystals, food, and for placing beneath potted plants (our orchid stands on 75mm cells and has bloomed continuously for the past year). Use on the body is not recommended because of the increased danger of breakage!

In comparison to the tachyon effect, the effect of the cell's color (frequency) accounts for only about three percent of the total. So be sure to select the colors that you like best, since you will then be certain to also use them.

Further Possibilities of Application

For injuries, include the cells in the last layers of the wrap (for example, a Tachyonized wrap). This also has a wonderful effect over a plaster cast. Place in the headband for meditation, concentration work, or when you have a headache. Use to charge water. Or simply sit on them when hemorrhoids plague you.

"Nutrition" Tip

An opal 24mm cell, with the round side stuck in the navel, helps in controlling all the processes connected with the digestive tract. As our most important source of survival when we were in the womb, our deepest themes of dependency and addiction are focused here. This is also helpful when fasting since the emotional component of food intake will then lose its influence. The navel cell has a useful application as an additional aid for gastrointestinal spasms, constipation or diarrhea, attacks of ravenous hunger, nausea, and flatulence.

From the Practice

One of my patients had suffered from an addiction to chocolate for years. Within two days of wearing the navel cell, her dependency completely disappeared. Totally amazed, she suddenly realized how dumb it was to have distributed chocolate and pralines everywhere in the house (even the cellar), so she could always nibble on them. With a feeling of disgust and liberation, she got rid of her entire supply. Her commentary: "If you knew what it means to me to be able to throw chocolate in the trash!"

Special Application Forms of Tachyonized Glass Cells

Cells for Correcting the Negative Effects of Cell Phones and Cordless Phones

Specially made square cells with adhesive foil are available for quick attachment to cell phones. The best place to stick them on is the backside of the device at the height of the loudspeaker, with the tachyon field through the cell phone in the direction of the head.

Chakra-Balancing Kits
(In the sizes 15mm, 24mm, and 30mm)

The word chakra is the Sanskrit name for "wheel." It signifies the main energy centers in the body, which are responsible for our various energy bodies. They manage the process of condensing the universal life energy and the development of consciousness. (For more details on understanding the chakras, also see the sections on the *Quality of One* on page 41 and the *Tachyon Personal Cocoon* on page 104). A balanced cooperation among all the chakras is an essential factor for harmonious development of consciousness. When the Tachyonized cells are applied to the corresponding places on the body, harmonizing universal life energy is guided directly into the chakras. This leads to harmonizing and strengthening the SOEFs of our physical, emotional, mental, and spiritual bodies. In turn, this is the precondition for experiencing unity with "All That Is".

The chakra journeys should take place in a peaceful, undisturbed ambiance and not last for more than 20 minutes at the beginning. A detailed description of such a journey is included in the Chakra Balancing Kit. Other methods for the work with the chakras can naturally have their effect potentiated by means of this aid.

Tachyonized Jewelry

Tachyonized glass cells and Tachyonized zirconiums are also available set in silver and gold in various colors and sizes. It's important to note that the clear and opal pieces also let the tachyons flow from the flat side, the zirconiums let them flow from the tips.

Pendants

According to their position, Tachyonized glass or zirconium pendants provide the throat chakra, the heart, and the thymus gland with balancing energy.

Background Information: Thymus Gland

The thymus gland lies directly beneath the sternum. Its functioning determines the quality of our immune system's performance. It is the training and information center for the essential defensive troops of our organism. In children and young people, it works at full speed; however, it gradually loses its performance capacity and mass in most adults. Western medicine pays no particular attention to this dynamic. However, in traditional Asiatic medicine, the maintenance and care of this gland plays a central role. Thousands of years of experience have shown the close correlation of the thymus-gland function with the maintenance of youthful energy up to an old age.

Further application recommendations: For all forms of heart and lung disorders, for general energizing, for children with chronic coughs, for colds and congestion (in addition to a lactalbumin-free diet.

The 30mm pendant can be worn above the solar plexus on a chain or cord of the corresponding length. Here it conducts balancing tachyon energy into the solar plexus and stomach, advisable for all forms of stomach disorders, as well as stress and stage fright.

Tachyonized Ear Studs

These are also available in various colors, forms, and two different sizes. Their opal glass cells also let the tachyon field flow from the flat side.

The most important effect of the ear studs is to synchronize the brain hemispheres.

Background Knowledge: Hemisphere Synchronization

The human cerebrum is divided into two separate processing centers. While the one half (hemisphere) tends to select the analytical-abstract path of processing information, the other hemisphere aims for a holistic-pictorial comprehension and classification. In a rhythm of about 90 minutes, the two sides alternate their dominance. Ingenious people have the ability to use both processing paths intertwined with each other or synchronously (at the same time). When there is a tremendous overemphasis upon a left-hemisphere, patriarchal lifestyle (analytical, abstract, and dominant), hardly any space remains for the talents related to the fine arts and intuition. This image of the outer world also finds a correlation in our brain in the form of left-brain hemisphere dominance, which can give many people a "headache."

Further effects are the stimulation of important reflex zones on the earlobe, which are related to the eye functions and the entire supply of energy to the head.

From the Practice: An editor I know responded to the question of whether or not she is familiar with tachyon as follows: "No! But two years ago I bought these ear studs at a trade fair." In response to my question as to whether they made a difference for her, she answered: "I didn't feel anything, but my migraines, from which I had suffered up to that time, disappeared."

Even fashion-conscious women who could fall back on a great treasure of ear jewelry, and are not even familiar with the theoretical background, no longer want to take off the ear studs. Sensitive ears hardly ever have infectious reactions to the ear studs because of the balancing tachyon field.

Tachyonized Animal Pendant Pet-Pouch

Either one or two 24mm tachyon cells can be placed in the small nylon bags on the collar of medium and large dogs. This provides an increased energy flow for our four-legged friends. When using these, please be sure that the energy flows out the flat side of the enclosed colored tachyon cells.

The dog tag and an address card also fit into these durable bags.

Report on Experience

Some people I know have a dog that was already suffering from old-age infirmity. It spent most of its time lying around and could no longer be interested in walking for any longer distances. A Pet-Pouch with two 24mm cells was put on its collar, dramatically changing the dog's behavior within a short time. The people are currently considering whether they should remove the cells since the dog energetically demands walks several times a day. Its reawakened, wild, and impetuous behavior is simply too much for them.

Flexcell 100

The Flexcell 100 is a special development of the Tachyonized silica disk. Completely flexible, unbreakable, and with a very dense, focused tachyon field, it is meant to be used for painful bodily disorders: slipped disks, lumbago, broken bones, and other injuries and conditions of pain.

Background Knowledge: Psychosomatic Medicine

In a large-scale study, 4000 cases of slipped disks were examined with the intention of finding out which of the occupational groups tended to develop this disorder. It was a great surprise to discover that there was absolutely no comprehensible correlation. The conclusion that resulted from this study: No physical strain or improper exertion can be the cause of this spinal-column complaint. Had the researchers been familiar with the model of the energetic continuum, they would presumably have more quickly reached the result that embellished their investigations after further research. The common factor that united 90 percent of all examined persons (such a percentage is considered highly significant in statistics), was an event in their lives, up to a maximum of two years before the slipped disk, that they couldn't bear. Among these were losing a job, deaths, divorces, and tragic occurrences that had remained undigested and that these people still carried around with them.

On the basis of these studies, we received scientifically founded evidence for the correlation of thoughts and feelings with physical disorders; in addition, they also gave us an indication of the maximum time before the idea of "I can't bear this!" manifests itself through the mental body, by way of the emotional body, into the physical form.

Report on Experience

The following case example illustrates how the healing process that tachyon stimulates also includes the emotional and mental level of our being.

A 46-year-old Russian immigrant, 196 centimeters (6'4") tall and with a friendly nature, dragged himself into my practice. For the last week, he had suffered from a slipped disk. He couldn't sit, could only lie down in one position, had hardly slept, his nerves were worn to a frazzle, and the medical treatment had hardly brought any relief. Six years ago, I had already treated him once for a similar situation. After seven treatments (which included injections, acupuncture, and chiropractic) we had achieved a complete freedom from complaints for these past six years. It wasn't possible to persuade him to clarify the background of this incident at that time. But now, after two tachyon applications (within three days of each other, between which he continuously wore the Flexcell 100) he was completely free of pain and could move without any problems. In addition, he quite spontaneously talked about his troubles at his place of work and fear of losing his job if he refused to do certain tasks. It was clear to him that things could not continue in this way, that he had already long crossed over the line. At the same time, he agreed that his fear was completely unfounded since he had certainly become indispensable to the company. This discussion took place without any psychotherapeutic guidance or intentions on my part. His healing occurred on all levels.

Construction of the Flexcell 100

The Flexcell 100 is made from six layers of latex alternating with silicon powder, poured into rubber, and then Tachyonized. The imprinted ATT logo shows the place from where the tachyon energy flows. In the accompanying belt, which is not Tachyonized, the Flexcell can be comfortably worn on any spot that requires a strong tachyon field.

The Flexcell is excellently suited for use on animals (particularly large ones like horses and cows) since it is large and strong, as well as easy to clean and disinfect.

Corresponding to the six layers of pulverized silicon disks, there is a six-fold tachyon density in comparison to a silicon disk. The length of the field is also 5 meters (5.5 yards), with dimensions of approx. 5" times 9". The variety of applications corresponds to those of the silica disks, in addition to the possibilities of using it directly on the body.

Many healers, massage therapists, and Reiki practitioners already use it as a type of "third hand," which they place on their patients' problem zones or wherever they have just worked. Other therapists wear it themselves during treatments and report that they have a distinctly increased flow of energy and protection from energy loss. Above all, this pertains when they work on extremely undercharged patients/clients.

For states of pain, wear the Flexcell continuously day and night (with the exception of bathing, showering, and making love). Once you are free of pain, continue for a few more days, depending on how long you have already had the pain. The explanation for this can be found under the topic of *Bifurcation* in the section on the TLC Bars.

Tip: If the circumstances prevent a suitable, graceful integration of the Flexcell into your wardrobe (office, place of work, mini-skirt), the Flexcell 100 can also be attached to the back of your chair at the level in which the disorder is located. You should naturally also pay attention to the direction in which the tachyon field is facing.

Happy Soles: Tachyonized Shoe Inserts

The Tachyonized shoe inserts are a wonderful aid for people who are on their feet much of the time. Homemakers, police officers, nurses, waiters and waitresses, salespeople...as well as athletes from joggers to top-performance athletes (including professional American basketball players) value the pleasant, harmonizing effect of Happy Souls.

The raw material for the surface is poron, which itself inhibits the growth of fungus and odor bacteria up to 90 percent. Because of the tachyon field, which extends to above the head, the supply of energy to the feet and entire leg area (including the pelvis) is also improved to a great extent. Many users no longer experience sweating and burning of the feet, even when they are on the move all day in their (work) shoes.

Because of the relieved energy congestion in the ankles and knees, there is a feeling of more contact with the ground while walking (grounding), combined with a feeling of "floating on clouds." Chilly legs become a thing of the past.

From the Practice

A client reported increased sweating of her feet since she began wearing the Tachyonized inserts. In addition, she experienced pain independent of whether she walked or moved. During the conversation, she remembered a long-forgotten torn ligament in her ankle, as well as the related healing process that had seemed to last an eternity. Ever since that time, she had always had cold feet. When the tachyon applications were intensified (glass cell attached, foot baths in warm water with Panther Juice, and Massage Cream), the complaints soon disappeared completely.

The owner of a natural foods store suffered from intense pain in the hips and knees. A chiropractic treatment brought just a minor amount of relief. The day that she attached the Happy Souls to her work slippers, the pain disappeared completely and no further treatment was necessary.

Wearing Happy Souls on a regular basis is particularly helpful because of their effect on the foot's *reflex zones*.

Background Knowledge: Reflex Zones

The few remaining medical records of the ancient Maya culture (Dresden Codex) handed down a complete therapy system for treating ailments through specific zones on the hands and feet. This is where our current widespread foot reflex-zone massage had its origins. Reflex zones are areas on the body surface that are connected with the interior through nervous and energetic connections. If, for example, the liver loses its state of balance and becomes ill, there is a reaction in the connected reflex zones on the right shoulder, on the foot soles, in the hands, in the nose, on the ears, in the eyes, on the liver meridian, and on the tongue. This may also be accompanied by hyperacidity and swelling of the tissue.

The pain caused by pressure or the changed tissue immediately shows the path back to the liver to the experienced diagnostician. Above all, the foot reflex zones react to a disorder of the organs connected with them by depositing salt crystals. When pressure is applied to these, the result is intense pain, which makes them a wonderful diagnostic field. Conversely, the dissolving of these types of disorders in the reflex zones through massage or pressure simultaneously leads to an increased flow of energy and dissolving of blockages in the corresponding afflicted organ.

Because of their effect on the foot reflex zones, wearing Tachyonized shoe inserts leads to an even, gentle harmonization of our entire inner life. When there is intense congestion in the feet, the regulation stimulated by the strengthened SOEFs can temporarily lead to an increase in foot sweating (detoxification) and to a sensation of heat.

Use of Happy Soles

Place into the footwear with the gray side facing up, and there you go! Attach with double-sided tape to sandals and slippers. If you must cut the soles down to size, use the remnants for some other purpose—like under plants!

Products with Gentle, Unfocused Tachyon Fields

Tachyonized silk and cotton is surrounded by a three-dimensional tachyon field that creates a gentle balancing on all levels. Above all, the large-scale SOEFs of the *emotional body* and the subtle areas of our energetic continuum respond to the application of these products. The raw materials are high quality and naturally washable. Hand washing is recommended to spare the materials.

Among the gentle, unfocused products are:
• headbands
• wristbands
• eye masks
• wraps
• joint hugs (elbows, knee joints, ankles)
• silk meditation wrap
• silk scarves.

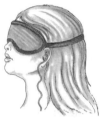

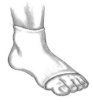

Tachyonized Headband

For all activities that require a high degree of concentration and mental clarity, this Tachyonized tool provides maximum service with a minimal effort. The harmonizing effect on all the areas of the various brain functions are in foremost here. While equilibrium in the cerebrum optimizes the above-mentioned mental abilities, balanced midbrain activities support a balanced emotional life. If the cerebellum functions to an optimal degree, it will produce graceful and appropriate patterns of movement. Finally, the brain stem makes sure that all systems important for survival (heartbeat, breathing, body temperature, etc.) are smoothly adapted to the necessary requirements. Above all, athletes value the even activation of these centers since increased fitness is immediately translated into improved results. Mental clarity, emotional balance, harmonious (energy-saving) patterns of motion, improved breathing, all of these factors support basic conditions for those who compete, as well as those who just want to enjoy life.

Likewise, I have been able to observe some dramatic improvements in schoolchildren with concentration disorders and dyslexia. The latter involves disturbed communication between the two brain hemispheres, which makes it difficult for children (as well as adults who suffer from it) to differentiate between left and right, for example. This results in stress-based errors when writing certain letters and their arrangement in words, so-called sloppy mistakes in math, as well as difficulties in learning foreign languages. Consequently, the children suffer from stress and anxious states before classes and because of ridicule from their fellow students. The consequences are the development of isolation and an injured sense of self-worth.

From the Practice

A 13-year-old girl came to my practice. She suffered from school stress, had bad grades in German (her native language) and math; despite her apparent intelligence, plans were being made to send her to a special school. Above all, she was very talented artistically and, like her parents and teachers, quite concerned about her own poor level of achievement at school. The path through numerous therapeutic facilities had brought no substantial improvement in her situation, but a unanimous diagnosis: dyslexia. With simple tests, I was able to determine disturbed communication between the two hemispheres of the cerebrum, which is considered one of the actual causes of dyslexia.

An essential component of the therapy was for her to wear a Tachyonized headband and wristbands, primarily while she did her homework. It would have been even better while in the classroom, but her vanity did not permit this. The next time she came to my practice, the girl reported that she had written the second-best math homework in her class. Her stress had disappeared, as had the worries of her parents and teachers, and she once again enjoyed learning. A further result was that she was able to reduce the number of errors in her essays so much that she had achieved the class average by the end of the year.

Her case was no exception in my practice. It very clearly showed me that the strategies suggested by her parents, teachers, and therapists for improving her performance had failed. This was because of their limited possibilities for promoting the brain's information processing in a harmonious and undisturbed manner. To the contrary, these attempts only increased the stress and accelerated her retreat into defiance and resignation. Only the constant harmonization of brain activity with the help of the Tachyonized aids broke the vicious circle and created the precondition for solving her problem.

Based on its wonderful effects of harmonizing brain function, it is understandable why the following users are also enthusiastic about the Tachyonized headband: the 95-year-old grandmother who studies the daily newspaper every morning, professional musicians, translators, oarsmen, authors, computer freaks, students, archers, "retired" ministers at prayer, mothers, people who meditate, joggers, drivers, tennis pros, headache-sufferers, people who have had strokes and head injuries, etc.

The Tachyonized headband can naturally also be worn around the neck when you are plagued by coughing, sore throat, and hoarseness; wear it on the arm or leg for pain and injuries; put it around potted plants, water bottles, fruit, crystals, dogs and cats, etc. The thinnest course participant I've had up to now even wore it around her waist as a belt!

Tachyonized headbands are made of cotton terry cloth in various colors and are available in two styles: the elastic stretch headband and the velcro headband. The second variation has a small, secret pocket. A maximum of three 24mm Tachyonized glass cells can be placed in them, which naturally has an immense intensifying effect through the focused tachyon field and is considered a secret tip among people who meditate (cosmic pocket-rocket).

Tachyonized Wristbands

Made of the same cotton terry cloth as the headband, the Tachyonized wristbands (pulse warmers) create a three-dimensional tachyon field. The gentle, balancing, and SOEF-energizing effect of these tools is recommended for use directly on site, primarily for handicraft activities and disorders in the areas of the hands and arms. On the other hand, they are also employed because of their remote action on our brain in the same situation, which is supported by the Tachyonized headband.

1. Improved functional capacity: The harmonizing and endurance-promoting effect of the Tachyonized wristbands is the reason for their frequent use by athletes of all disciplines, including tennis, rowing, weight-lifting, handball...(even for chess, which becomes clear under point 3). However, others who can profit from it are artisans, musicians, secretaries, programmers, homemakers, drivers, sculptors, massage therapists, Reiki practitioners, healers, geriatric nurses...in short, people who physically strains their hands and arms, as well as those who are dependent upon a skillful, finely-tuned coordination of their actions.

2. Observed health-promoting effects: In cases of the carpal tunnel syndrome (in connection with Panther Juice and Tachyonized glass cells), tennis elbow, all forms of joint complaints, tensions and spasms, injuries, shoulder-hand syndrome, and circulation disorders (cold hands), among other things.

Studies of blood under the dark-field microscope have impressively proved the fascinating effect of tachyons on the quality of the red blood corpuscles. Both the oxygen reception and the flexibility of the cell walls increases (rouleaux disappear!), which explains one aspect of the endurance-increasing effect of the Tachyonized wristbands.

3. Effect on the brain: By energizing the corresponding acupuncture points and nerve paths, there is a harmonization of the brain hemispheres, similar to that of the Tachyonized headbands and Tachyonized ear studs. The wristbands also develop their effect in support of mental clarity, concentration, and memory for the above-mentioned groups of people, as well as for schoolchildren (dyslexia), students, authors, and everyone who performs mental work.

From the Practice

A master piano-builder told me that since he has been wearing the Tachyonized wristbands while tuning pianos, he no longer has had tension and pain in his shoulders and arms at night. Furthermore, since he started doing this, he requires a significantly shorter amount of time to bring the pianos into the best tuning. One of the reasons for this was his increased concentration. But his considerably improved sense of hearing plays an even larger role. When you are in tune yourself, tuning an instrument is probably easier. He knew that he wasn't just imagining this because of the difference he noticed whenever he *didn't* wear the Tachyonized wristbands at work.

Tachyonized Eye Masks

This Tachyonized eye mask, which is covered with silk, is a wonderful help for people who have difficulty in falling asleep. The gentle, balancing effect on the activity of the cerebrum, the eye muscles, and a large number of important acupuncture points around the eyes is the reason that the eye mask renders its service both when a person sleeps too much and when there are sleep disorders.

Since it is weaker than the Tachyonized eye pillow, the eye mask has the advantage that it can be used in positions other than prone. It has become an important companion for many people who travel by plane and train since it can also lead to deep relaxation and restful sleep in such environments.

The eye mask is also an important aid for occasional short breaks, whether on long trips in the car or at work. I have given more detail on the essential significance of 20-minute breaks, during which the body can completely recuperate itself, in the description of the *Tachyon Personal Cocoon*. (See page 104)

The effects of the Tachyonized eye mask mentioned above also facilitate the path to deep meditation.

Additional Information: Meditation

Meditation is the state in which we are merged with All That Is, free of any activity, of personal desiring and striving, of ideas and thoughts. We yield ourselves to the inexhaustible flow of universal life energy. We are one with God and the world. We are timeless and weightless... Meditation can be equated with spiritual realization, with "coming home," with the development of our highest potential as conscious beings. This state of being is not bound to any conditions in the outside world. The declared goal of most spiritual traditions is to live life in a state of continuous meditation—not just when sitting still, on Sunday morning, or on a retreat at the feet of someone who is a master of this state.

Within this context it is important to not confuse the path to meditation with the actual state. Breathing and physical exercises are important aids on the path to unity since they make it possible for the energies of all our body levels to start flowing. The same applies to mental exercises, prayers, contemplation, mantras, and singing. The contents are only as good and useful as they support us in "waking up" to the state of meditation. Their significance is limited to the phase in which they get us flying and bring us to sweet merging with our divine essence. By being conscious of the framework in which the "meditation techniques" (spiritual paths, systems of belief, and religions with the corresponding practices) develop their role, we can recognize all the ideas that separate us from the whole to be pure superficialities. Then the trumpets no longer fight against the violins in the immense variety of our human orchestra on this planet, nor does the triangle rebel against the superior strength of the bass drums. The mutual song in consciousness creates a new level of playing together, of joy and unity, for the variety of instruments.

Tachyonized Wraps

These Tachyonized elastic wraps are made of superior raw material, which gives them a long-term durability with a high level of quality. The velcro fastener saves on bothersome taping or pinning. The three-dimensional tachyon field surrounding the wrapped zone at an angle of 360 degrees provides the optimal supply to SOEFs that have been disturbed by the injury.

The main area of application for this Tachyonized tool is therefore all forms of injuries on the arms, legs, and joints, as well as bruises, sprains, broken bones (wrap over the plaster cast in this case), and cuts and scrapes. The possibility of including Tachyonized glass cells in the wound material potentiates the effectiveness many times over. I have seen some cases of deep cuts treated in this way that have healed without pain and scars.

In many cases of chronic joint complaints, such as arthritis or gout, the Tachyonized wrap coupled with other necessary healing steps has led to relief from pain.

This can also be an indispensable component in healing and caring for animals, particularly racehorses and riding animals.

Background Knowledge: X-Rays and Pain

A large-scale evaluation of X-ray photographs in relation to the assessed pain findings has resulted in an astonishing discovery: The hit accuracy of an x-ray picture to determine whether the respective patient has pain or does not have pain was only 40 percent, even when there were seriously pathological changes in the joints. This means it is highly unscientific to relate pain in the locomotor system with a x-ray picture. As a result, pain can be experienced in a completely inconspicuous X-ray finding, and no pain may be experienced in a finding that is evaluated as highly pathological. This unexpected result sent the research team off to search for the true causes for states of pain.

The results of their years of strict scientifically conducted studies: In about 98 percent of the cases of pain in the locomotion system (back, joints, etc.) chronically cramped musculature plays the triggering role. They furnished the proof of their theory by means of a therapy that once again activated the corresponding, frequently encapsulated, muscles in a simple manner, achieving freedom from pain. With this scientific work, which unfortunately has not found the appropriate entry to established orthopedics, all "verdicts" of lifelong pain on the basis of a pathological finding by means of radiological examination have been suspended. The path for further efforts toward health and freedom from pain is once again open.

The wraps, available in four different widths, should not be missing in any home first-aid kit or sports bag.

Tachyonized Hugs

People who don't like to use wraps have the Tachyonized hugs (for ankles, elbows, hands, and knees) available to them as a wonderful aid. In this simple and effective way, they can use the 360-degree effect of a gentle, three-dimensional tachyon field for their joints. These are applied for existing pain and complaints, as well as to simply protect joints that are intensely strained on the job or during sports.

Background Knowledge: Toxin Management

When the body doesn't succeed in eliminating the occurring toxins through the regulated, designated paths, the following multi-level emergency program is employed:

1. Removing the toxins from the blood circulation to the intercellular tissue. Here they lead to overacidity, which must be deactivated through connective tissue. The results are swollen cutaneous areas and muscle fiber that is stuck together.
2. Excretion through the mucous membranes of the respiratory tract. These toxins subsequently provoke the production of mucous. With its help, the body can then excrete them. Manifestation forms of this level are colds and sinusitis, as well as bronchitis and bronchial asthma in protracted and difficult cases.
3. According to the constitution type, the body then also attempts to take the path through the skin and causes symptoms such as rashes (neurodermatitis), pus pimples, furuncles, and open wounds that do not heal.
4. If all these ways of disposing of poisons are inadequate, the organism then stores toxins in the parts of our bodies that have the least metabolism. Above all, this means our cartilage and joints. In this "final disposal" stage, a process develops that ends up in the destruction of these tissue layers. We can find this described in the forms of rheumatism.

Experience has shown that simply reacting to the symptoms accompanying our body's management of toxins without eliminating the background leads to a continuous worsening of these symptoms. The use of Tachyon Energy for joint trouble leads, through strengthening the SOEFs, to the corresponding detoxification possibilities in the cartilage, intercellular tissue, and muscle cells. It therefore contributes to helping eliminate the basis of the above-mentioned symptoms from the body. In keeping with the sluggishness of the metabolism in these regions, spontaneous healing tends to be rare. The slow progress of improvement is natural and shouldn't discourage users, causing them to doubt the effectiveness of tachyon. Those afflicted with this disorder should also avoid the additional influx of toxins and support the self-healing powers of the organism through the appropriate diet and supply of water.

There are currently hugs for ankles and elbows (available in three sizes) and knees (available in four sizes). The effectiveness of application can also be greatly increased here by adding Tachyonized glass cells. Hand hugs, specifically intended for gout and joint inflammations of the finger and hand joints, are also available in two sizes.

Tachyonized Silk Meditation Wrap

The most popular tachyon tool is probably the Tachyonized silk meditation wrap. The reason for this may be because the gentle and extensive harmonization opens the emotional body in particular for these sensations. When we are wrapped in it like a loving hug, emotional blockages and imbalances melt away like ice in the sun. The mind becomes calm and clear.

Above all, using the Tachyonized silk meditation wrap after deep emotional work in connection with healing work or therapy shortens the integration time to a few minutes, as opposed to the hours that usually occupy the client (and therapist). Actors and musicians, as well as anyone else who must deal with stage fright and nervousness, can put the balancing effect of this dream made of silk to great use before performing.

Placed in the cradle and baby carriage of newborns and infants, the wrap protects against disharmonious patterns from the surrounding world, such as electrosmog and other people's imbalanced emotions. It also makes it easier for them to cope with life in their bodies, which is quite strenuous at the start. The result is a greater degree of contentment, less crying, and sleep that is deeper, longer, and therefore more restful. This cuddly blanket is excellent for the promotion of balanced development.

The Tachyonized silk meditation wrap naturally also enormously improves sleep quality for adults; for example, between the top sheet and the normal blanket. It soothes the disruption of the entire energy field by intense emotionally colored dream experiences. It optimizes and accelerates dream processing, contributing to sleep with an increased recuperation value.

For all health disorders with a strong emotional context, the silk wrap offers great additional advantages. These disorders include asthma, allergies, skin rashes, gastric ulcers, spasms, exhaustion syndromes, and depressions, as well as conditions after accidents, operations, fever, and all childhood diseases.

From the Practice

At an information evening in my practice on the topic of self-help with Tachyon Energy, there was a woman who had suffered from severe bronchial asthma for years. She was gray in the face, short of breath, and in a general state of poor health. Without any particular intentions, I offered her a silk meditation wrap, which she then kept around her for the rest of the evening. To her own astonishment, she didn't need any asthma remedy the entire evening, although she had come in the middle of an asthma attack for which she usually would have had to spray every half an hour. But the change in this woman's entire charisma was the most fascinating event of the evening: rosy cheeks, a relaxed and friendly smile on a face previously dominated by an expression of fear and doubt. To my great surprise, I never saw this woman again. This distinct experience did not lead her to take the next step, at least not in my practice, for a possible healing.

There have also been good experiences with the Tachyonized silk meditation wrap in facilities for the care of mentally handicapped people. Above all, this has helped in working with autistic children, who are otherwise hardly accessible.

However, people who have recognized the blessings of meditation for their personal development are the largest group of users. Wearing the wrap during meditation creates a space of deep peace and greatest balance, relaxes the body, and calms the mind. These are all preconditions for the experience of unity with All That Is.

Tachyonized Silk Scarf

Everything that I have written about the Tachyonized silk wraps also applies, in a correspondingly lesser degree, to the Tachyonized silk scarves. As an accessory, they can even be inconspicuously worn with a more formal wardrobe. Above all, they are a wonderful aid for people who use their voice and self-expression to present themselves in the limelight of public attention. The SOEFs in the throat area, which can "leave someone speechless" when excited or agitated, are gently balanced and energized, something that singers, musicians, and speakers value to an equal degree.

For all forms of disturbances in the area of the throat, the heart, and the respiratory tract, the Tachyonized silk scarf provides additional help. Used as a headband, it promotes the ability to concentrate and the synchronization of the hemispheres. If no Tachyonized wrap is at hand, a scarf can also naturally serve as a source of tachyon over an injured area.

The same care recommendations apply for the Tachyonized silk products as for conventional silk. Even if the traces of time have made them unattractive at some point, the subatomic restructuring through the Tachyonization process is maintained without restriction. Such pieces can, for example, be sewed into clothing, wrapped around drinking glasses to charge water, woven into plants to strengthen their SOEFs with tachyons. You can make little bags out of them for carrying and preserving your gemstones and jewelry, or use them to carry snacks such as apples. Wear them as a hairband, sew them into your pillowcase, or wrap them around the dog's collar. There are countless possibilities waiting to be translated into action.

A Tachyonized tool never stops serving!

Products with Strong, Unfocused 3-D Tachyon Fields

These Tachyonized tools impart a strong, three-dimensional tachyon field that permits both intensive and large-scale applications. Just as the dense layers of our physical body react to the density of the tachyon field with quicker balancing, the broad application also simultaneously energizes the superordinate SOEFs of the emotional and mental areas.

Among the strong, unfocussed 3-D products are:
• Sleep Pad
• Life-Padd
• Vitalizer II
• eye pillow
• neck pillow
• animal pendant Life-Capsule.

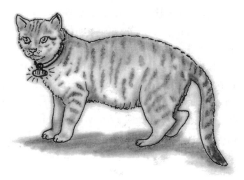

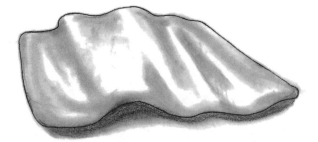

Tachyonized Sleep Pad

The raw material for this superlative product is a specially developed fabric of aero silicon fibers. As applies to all silicon compounds, when Tachyonized this substance develops a strong antenna effect for tachyon. The material was first used in the Life-Padd, the Vitalizer II, and the Cocoon strips. Constantly developing advancement in the technology of Tachyonization now permits the production of such large, intensive-effect tools at lower prices. The extraordinary intensity of the balancing tachyon field, which has a simultaneous effect on the entire organism (all SOEFs) because of the size of the blanket, opens a new level for the use of Tachyon Energy: healing and development during sleep!

Background Knowledge: Sleeping Periods

Do you know how much of our lifetime we spend in the state of sleep? Let me quickly calculate it: At an average of eight hours of sleep per night, which incidentally is one third of our lifetime, we sleep 240 hours in a month with 30 days. That's 2,920 hours per year, which would be somewhat more than 120 days if they were uninterrupted!

Most people only recognize the immense importance of sleep for well-being, health, and ultimately, survival, when they experience a lack of it. Today we know the medical background for the meaning of sleep, how the body cleanses and renews itself during this time, fills up the supply areas in the glands and nervous system, and stores energy in the form of glycogen (storage form of the blood sugar). Only this makes a functioning metabolism possible the next day. We know about the processing of emotional and mental themes during the dream phase of sleep and its essential significance for our emotional/mental state. We know all of this, as well as the numerous influences that can promote or disrupt these processes.

It would fill many volumes of books to make room for exhaustive information on this subject, including the resulting advice for appropriate behavior to support it. This is not my calling, so I'd like to make it much easier on myself. Let me simply describe what the Tachyonized Sleep Pad does for me when I sleep on it:

1. It surrounds me with a strong tachyon field, which harmonizes harmful and dissonant frequencies from the outside such as earth

rays, electrosmog, weather-caused atmospheric energy fields (such as spherics), "spirits," etc.). This supports me during a phase in which my energy system is more open and vulnerable for these types of influences than in the waking state.

2. The energizing effect of tachyons on my entire-body SOEF allows it to regulate, with the purpose of balancing, the entire subordinate SOEFs of organ systems, organs, cells, molecules, atoms, down to the corresponding pions. The effect is an even, harmonious increase of all body energies, smoothly functioning regeneration work, improved metabolic efficiency, an undisturbed immersion in the deep sleep phases, a quicker processing of stress, and generally more restful sleep.

This is an optimal possibility for taking care of ourselves and supporting our healing, health, and development during the very important periods of sleep. However, the first nights on a Tachyonized Sleep Pad can also bring moving experiences with them. To the degree in which the SOEFs want to create the state of optimal balance, all types of detoxification reactions may occur. Users report experiencing nightly outbreaks of sweat, colorful and intensive dream experiences, states of unrest with frequent waking, ranging up to difficulties in falling asleep that are similar to how they react when they drink coffee. On the other hand, others joyfully experience falling asleep immediately. They have restful nights from the very beginning and increased energy during the entire next day.

This is always an individual balancing process, controlled by the current needs and possibilities of the regulating SOEFs. If you have undesired reactions, I suggest slowly getting used to it in the form of lying on the pad for just an hour or two at one time. After several nights, the excessive reactions will disappear, making way for gentle and constant harmonization.

There are naturally enough other application possibilities for the Tachyonized Sleep Pad during the day as well, in addition to sleeping on it. Above all, it can be used by seriously ill people whose vital energy stagnates more and more because they can only lie in bed without much movement or for those who want to recover more quickly after illnesses.

On the treatment lounge for all types of healing practitioners, massage therapists, and physiotherapists, the strong tachyon field facilitates a deep opening for this kind of work. It also supports quick integration of all physical, emotional, and mental movements that are triggered during the treatment. The strong balancing effect naturally also affects the person giving the treatment. It protects against the otherwise unavoidable energy decrease caused by absorbing the patients' dissonant energy patterns. All processes take place more quickly and in a more balanced manner, which gives the person being treated a more intensive and distinct experience.

Related to the use of the Tachyonized Sleep Pad for meditation, the term "flying carpet" most closely describes the possible experiences. The everyday "obligatory act," with its mental carousels, feelings of reluctance, painful back and sore knees, and all the adversities that can complicate the path into silence, becomes a time of lightness, depth, and clarity through the nourishing tachyon field. Like an energy egg, it helps the person inside it defy the laws of gravity. Body exercises like yoga and Qi Gong, breathing techniques, contemplation, and prayer experience a wonderful deepening of their effect on this Sleep Pad.

The Tachyonized Sleep Pad on the seat of the car finally puts an end to tense backs and tiredness while driving. As a long-distance driver, these symptoms have shown me the frequently undesired limitations. The recuperation phase during the rest that I now need less frequently is more intensive and shorter. The state of my energy at the destination is not much different than when I left and the aggravation phases because of the imbalanced behavior of my traffic colleagues are clearly shorter. All in all, driving long distances has become less difficult and safer because of the evenly high level of concentration. My seventh sense for radar traps has improved as well!

Life-Padd (Tachyonized Cushion)

The Tachyonized cushion is the mini-version of the Sleep Pad. The core of the cushion is a Tachyonized fabric made of aero silicon fibers, as in the Sleep Pad, which is sewed into a special nylon material. In this case, nylon is the material of choice since the silicon fibers cannot pierce through this dense nylon fabric. It also provides enough firmness to maintain the form. This core is put into a robust, washable sleeve with nylon on the underside and fleece on the top side. A foam insert provides makes it soft and comfortable to sit on.

Above all, the strong three-dimensional tachyon field energizes the SOEFs in the pelvic and abdominal area of the person sitting on the cushion. This, in turn, leads to an improved supply of energy to the spinal column and back. The Life-Padd provides wonderful service for all disorders in the area of the bladder, the reproductive organs (such as menstrual complaints and prostatism), for digestive disorders, hemorrhoids, hip disease, and complaints in the lower portion of the back.

Originally meant as support for people in wheelchairs, it has now found many other fans, especially among professional sitters like secretaries, public officials, drivers, and students—and moviegoers!

The easily removable tachyon core can also be placed under the sheets, where it develops the harmonizing, healing, and supportive effect for the ill. It can also be placed into the cradle of infants or used on the treatment table. There are no limits to the possibilities.

This cushion always accompanies me while walking in the woods with my dog, allowing me to sit comfortably, dry, and energized next to my favorite trees and just enjoy the day or meditate.

The cushion has also found widespread use as a pad for cats and dogs. While the latter appreciate the balancing effect of the tachyons without exception, cats appear to have rather mixed feelings toward this ordering energy, unless they are ill. I have heard the most adventurous stories on the topic of cats and tachyon, all of which allow the conclusion that these furry four-legged creatures have a distinct, highly individualized emotional nature.

Vitalizer II Belt

The Tachyonized Vitalizer II belt is made of cotton and, like the Life-Padd, it has a core of aero silicon fiber—but here it is sewn into it. The aero silicon fiber is a special development of astronautics and not related to glass fibers or similar materials, which are said to be a health hazard. Through the Tachyonization process, this belt is available to us as a tachyon antenna that completely surrounds the body and energizes all the SOEFs of the pelvic and abdominal area.

Background Knowledge: Zones of Power

The belt was considered a symbol of power in ancient times. It was reserved for rulers and other powerful people. We find the energetic reality behind this "symbol" described in the shamanic tradition, as well as in Traditional Chinese Medicine. Zones and points that connect the lower with the upper body border the region of the belt. These direct the root's vital power to the crown, filling our entire organism with liveliness and power in the process. Whether it is called the "belt vessel" in Chinese Medicine or the "shaman belt" in various other traditions, physical strength and health are directly related to a permeable and energetic functioning of these zones.

This also explains the name of the Vitalizer II belt, which is based on many people's experiences of its life-giving qualities. Particularly healers who work with direct energy transference value how it intensifies the energy flow and increases the effectiveness of their healing work. At the same time, the tachyon field protects people from negative energy patterns. Athletes are pleased about the additional energy and endurance, as well as homemakers and mothers who have similar demands placed on them in experiencing the limits of their capabilities. It is ideal for pregnancy and the period of regeneration after birth, as well as for the energy-demanding phase of breastfeeding with its sleepless nights. For bellies with a circumference greater than 38 inches (not only during pregnancy), there is an extension of this belt that can also be used for the Flexcell 100.

For disorders in the area of the inner organs (such as constipation, gastric ulcers, kidney stones, and gallbladder disease), the Vitalizer II should be favored over the Flexcell 100 because of its gentler and more comprehensive effect on the regulation of SOEFs. This also applies to certain forms of menstrual complaints, especially those with a strong emotional context. In these cases, the Vitalizer II should be worn continuously, even at night.

Like all Tachyonized tools, the Vitalizer II belt should be used as much and as creatively as possible. It can naturally be worn on both sides and wrapped around injured or tired legs and arms. Use it to crown an aching head or bathe the chest or upper back in a tachyon field by wearing it as a sash. Attach it to the back of your chair at any desired height to relieve pain or promote relaxation. It can be wrapped around water bottles and the pots of sick plants, as well as placed into the dog basket.

Tachyonized Eye Pillow

About 200 grams of Tachyonized glass beads, sewed into a little bag of pure, high-quality silk, make this eye pillow a very popular all-round talent. Its special feature is that the individual little glass beads are directional, meaning that they are Tachyonized to be focused. The result is that they emit a strong, concentrated tachyon field. Distributed zigzag in the little bag, they in turn create a three-dimensional field. This means that the eye pillow combines the strong, balancing potency of focused products with the effectiveness of the three-dimension tools.

As the name implies, the eye pillow is primarily meant to be placed on the eyes. Even after a short time, a pleasant relaxation begins here. Then it stretches across the entire head, neck, and shoulder area and ultimately—usually within 10 to 15 minutes—extends to the entire body. The dissolving of blockages in the eye area is equivalent to letting go of control and will, our active mental functions that are oriented toward the outside world and usually over-emphasized. Of the many levels that we reach by applying the eye pillow—like important acupuncture points, the fine musculature of the eyes, nose reflex zones, frontal and paranasal sinuses—I would like to single out an especially important one that only recently has been researched and published for medical experts.

Background Knowledge: Light and Brain Activity

In a study related to the effect of sunlight on us human beings, researchers from the specialized area of psychoneuroimmunoendocrinology (memorize this word and impress your friends!) came to the following conclusion: Only with at least 20 minutes of midday sunlight every day, directly(!) on the retina of the eyes, can the most important brain glands and centers responsible for the smooth functioning of the defensive system (...immuno...), the hormone system (...endocrino...), the autonomic nervous system (...neuro...), and therefore our sense of well-being (...psycho...) adequately fulfill these tasks. Less than 20 minutes will eventually lead to a loss of vitality in one, two, or three of these basic support systems of our bodily functions. The consequences are lowered resistance, all types of hormonal disorders, stress, and, above all, depression.

Experiments done on patients during this study concerning depressions that had been untreatable up to that point caused the depressions to disappear in almost 30 percent of the study participants. Who hasn't experienced the winter depression that lets us yearn for the springtime sun or urges us to go to the travel agency and book a place in the sun somewhere? Presumably a relic from the ages of winter sleep, this dynamic not only gets to us in winter but also during longer periods of bad weather in the summer.

Translated into our model, this means: The SOEFs that control the retina require highly charged SOEFs from the sun in order to activate the corresponding nerve SOEFs. In turn, these report what is happening in the outside world to the control centers. As a result, our entire organism is attuned to this activity. A lack of sun SOEFs equals not wanting to do anything!

The outstanding effect of the Tachyonized eye pillow is therefore found in its ability to energize the retina SOEFs like the sun, sending the above-mentioned control centers the signal that the light is green and the coast is clear. Incidentally, these control centers are the pituitary gland, the pineal gland, and the hypothalamus, which we will encounter in numerous other places in this book. This is no wonder since these are the top floors of our most important bodily functions.

When placed on the eyes, the Tachyonized eye pillow is an important component of the *Tachyon Personal Cocoon*. It should also be mentioned here that if you have intraocular pressure or sensitive eyes in general, the glass beads should be moved to the side to avoid unnecessary pressure on the eyeball.

From the Practice

A patient of mine was to be fitted for glasses since the doctor had diagnosed extensive disorders in her eyes. She called me with the question of whether the Tachyon Personal Cocoon could help her eye problems since she would rather invest her money in tachyons than in a pair of glasses. Since I am always careful about how I answer such questions, I briefly explained to her the expected effect of the tachyon fields: what may occur around the eye and in the eye is ultimately up to the discretion of the corresponding SOEFs. Full of trust in her SOEFs, she bought the Personal Cocoon (accompanied by the skepticism of her husband, a physicist) and laid in it on a regular basis while her spouse and daughter made light of her.

Fourteen days later, she had another appointment with the ophthalmologist, who could detect none(!) of the previously diagnosed findings. Since she didn't want to tell him about the Personal Cocoon and tachyons, he was simply astonished since such a normalization (healing) could not have been expected considering the intensity of the disorders, particularly not within such a short period of time.

The versatility of the Tachyonized eye pillow explains its popularity: place it on your neck and shoulders or on painful joints, sit on it while meditating, lay it on your head, knead it in your hands (reflex zones), or put it into the baby's bed. You can also place the Tachyonized glass beads in a little toy dolphin, turtle, or frog normally filled with rice or sand and make a child happy on the outside and inside.

Tachyonized Neck Pillows

The Tachyonized neck pillow is a typical example for the development of the Tachyonized tools presented in this book. The thing that all these aids have in common is the conveyance of tachyons, so each of them can be used for everything. Only the practical aspect in terms of effectiveness and the type of application accelerates the progress of continual new product development. In the case of the neck pillow, the question about a tool that could be helpful and simple to use for stress was the trigger.

A typical, widespread stress pattern, as it manifests itself in our physical body, looks like this: tense neck and shoulder muscles, blockages in the gallbladder meridian in this sector, disturbed outflow of lymph from the head, and the tendency toward pressure headaches, up to the point of migraines. Since stress also directly affects the stomach, we find blockages in the corresponding stomach meridians. The energy flow through the spinal column is reduced because of the congestion at the beginning of the cervical spine, which leads to concentration disorders and tiring too quickly. The longer this pattern is maintained, the more symptoms accumulate. These range from the unpleasant to those that produce illness.

The solution to this problem must also be simple since the people who tend to have such a stress pattern usually don't tolerate any protracted, complicated, and costly aids and measures. The solution is a neck pillow, adapted precisely to these symptoms with thousands of Tachyonized glass beads (about twice as much as in the eye pillow). Just like the eye pillow, the neck pillow combines the advantages of a strongly focused tachyon field with those of a comprehensively effective three-dimensional product. On both sides, it covers points on the stomach meridian, the most important gallbladder point for supplying the head and shoulders, and the corresponding lymph points for improving the outflow from the head. It crosses the neck at a point that plays a significant role for the energy flow in the spinal column. This all vividly describes the wonderfully relaxing effect, even shortly after the neck pillow has been applied. And it is also very easy to use. It can be placed inconspicuously beneath the jacket or on top of it. It can be taken off or applied quickly, making it ideal for the office and the manager level, where most people afflicted by this problem can be found.

Further examples of application: placed on the chakras of the front center line of the body, inserted into the belt loops of pants, or positioned in front of the keys of the keyboard. Or, as in my case at the moment while I write, put the Neck Pillow in front of the computer notebook with your wrists on it to prevent cramping of the fingers, wrists, and the rest of the arm. This prevents the feared carpal tunnel syndrome and brings to light bright ideas through the harmonization of the brain hemispheres.

Tachyonized Animal Pendant Life-Capsule

Life-Capsule animal pendants are filled with little Tachyonized glass beads. They are available in two sizes: the smaller of the two is meant for little pets like cats, hares, and rabbits. The larger is excellently suited for dogs of all sizes and goats. Since our four-legged friends are usually well-integrated in their energetic continuum, the tachyon products achieve a quick balancing of disorders and diseases with a minimum of effort. The Tachyonized animal pendants represent an effective means of preventing illness and maintaining the health of pets.

Incidentally: As a keychain pendant, the Life-Capsule is an exclusive gift for friends.

From the Animal Practice

An aged pinscher had suffered for years from fatty tumors that be-came infected time and again. These complaints could not be influ-enced by any type of veterinarian measures. Although the possibil-ity of an operative procedure was taken into consideration, the age of the dog prevented this. A Tachyonized Life-Capsule was the only measure that led to the fatty tumors disappearing completely within two weeks. Intended solely for strengthening the general vitality, the tachyons made it possible for the dog to heal its tumors com-pletely and permanently.

Products for External Application on the Skin

The spectrum of this product series extends from skin care to a great variety of disruptive patterns of the skin, muscles, and joints. It should be taken into special consideration here that certain skin areas (such as the reflex zones, dermatome, acupuncture points, etc.) are closely connected with the interior of the body and therefore represent gateways through which we can reach the entire organism. In addition, there is also the possibility of gently harmonizing larger areas of the body.

Only the purest quality raw materials are used for Tachyon products. These have also been selected according to ecological aspects. Animal products are not used, and no type of animal testing is carried out or promoted in any way!

Among the products for outer application are:
• Panther Juice
• Ultra-Balance Massage Oil
• Ultra-Balance Massage Cream
• Ultra-Freeze, Passion Dew
• Tach-O-Vera
• Retinyl Gel
• Ultra Pure Vitamin A Cream
• Ultra Pure Vitamin E Cream.

Tachyonized Panther Juice

Before this Tachyonized skin oil became available for public sale, its effects were studied in 22 practices. The three years of development time were worth it: In over 90 percent of the cases in which Panther Juice was used in connection with other tachyon tools, it was possible to observe a significant reduction (75 percent and more) or a complete disappearance of the pain. These results have now been confirmed throughout the world.

The Unique Composition

Vitamin-B complex (source of the characteristic "panther" smell), Vitamin E, folic acid, magnesium citrate, zinc and manganese (as a chelate), selenium, aloe vera, arnica oil, peppermint oil, and others.

The composition of these individual vitamins, minerals, and plant components has been selected so that they quickly penetrate the skin into the deep tissue and muscle layers, strengthening the SOEFs at the molecular and cellular level. This initiates a harmonization process, causing cleansing work to occur and an improved metabolism in the corresponding areas. Within about 20 minutes, the body processes the greater portion of the components and excretes the unused excesses through the kidneys. This can result in urine that has an intensely yellow to brown coloring! What remains is an optimally prepared field where the body can complete its additional healing work.

Background Knowledge: Cell Environment and Basic Regulation

We have the research of Dr. Pischinger at the University of Vienna, Austria, to thank for deep insights into the interplay between cells and their environment. He has described how directly the state of the environment around our cells influences their functioning. Like passing through a swamp, nutrients wander from the blood vessels into the cells and waste products from the cell metabolism take the reverse path. The organism controls this exchange through the nerve cells, which lead directly into this intercellular substance. It also controls the hormones and other messenger substances by letting the swamp become denser or lighter. The most important defensive achievements of our immune system take place in this area between the cells. Wastes in the form of acids are stored temporarily to keep the blood clean. All of the reconstruction work for injured or destroyed tissue occurs here as well. If acids are stored in this area—for example, after injuries or because of stress and false nutrition—a vicious circle begins that can end in the functional impairment of more or less large areas of tissue.

Try pinching the top layer of your outer upper arm between your fingers. If this hurts and isn't possible, then the tissue is presumably swollen as a result of deposits in the form of acids. This reduces the supplying of the cells with the necessary nutrients, just as it decreases the removal of wastes, leading to additional acids that cause the tissue to swell even more. The swamp becomes increasingly impenetrable in both directions. The cells cut off from the supply suffer a deficiency, no longer maintaining the performance required for smooth functioning. If this process takes place beneath the threshold of pain, we accept it as natural and call it "aging." However, it usually does bring pain and disease with it.

Almost every chronic illness—such as those associated with rheumatism, allergies, neurodermatitis, vascular sclerosis, etc.—can only arise on the basis of intercellular tissue that has already been disturbed. Eighty percent of all pain conditions in "civilized" countries affect the locomotor system, costing billions in public funds. This pain reveals the final stage of body's regulative ability in the corresponding tissue sections. It also means that the body's capitulation to an excess of acids that can no longer be neutralized and excreted. A painful destructive process of the physical form is initiated as a result. Since this process affects the intercellular tissue of the entire organism and not just the part of it that hurts, successfully treating the localized pain lulls the patient into a false sense of security. Only when we cleanse all the cells and the intercellular tissue of blocked toxins or acids, as well as switching to live food and a lively lifestyle, can we create the precondition for true healing.

Application

With this background, the limits and possibilities of using Panther Juice (PJ) in particular become clear. If the fantastic effect of this Tachyonized skin oil isn't accompanied by the above measures necessary for a lasting healing process, the desired result will remain inadequate. I therefore recommend that the pain-reducing effect of Tachyonized Panther Juice be used on anyone suffering from rheumatism, arthrosis (degenerative joint disease), gout, and other chronic states of pain to take a new approach to changing disease-causing lifestyles in the sense of the above-mentioned ideas.

All of this also explains why very different reactions to the application of Tachyon Energy can be observed. When pain arises where there was no pain before, this may mean that the immobilized acid deposits are being dissolved. In this process, the sensitivity of the nerves increases or tissue helps itself by increasing the temperature (inflammation). In this case, treat the afflicted pain zones, drink plenty of water (1.5 to 2 liters/quarts a day), and possibly reduce the extent of the tachyon application. But don't stop completely (see the topic of *Bifurcation* in the section on TLC Bars, page 114).

Above all, in the area of the joints, where a very slow metabolism takes place and strong toxins may possibly be stored, the healing process may occur more slowly. It may draw itself out over weeks and months. However, in almost every case, we can expect a distinct reduction of pain within 15 minutes.

Panther Juice is an essential component of a strategy for applying tachyons in conditions of pain. This strategy is imparted in the *Tachyon Practitioner Training* and used around the world with great success by professional healing practitioners, as well as interested laypeople.

In addition to its application for pain of the musculature, tissue, and joints in the area of chronic diseases, Panther Juice also helps against acne, furuncles, circulatory disturbances (in addition, stop smoking and eating meat), sport injuries, sprains, bruises, inflammations, closed skin diseases, insect bites, and sunburn(!).

From the Practice

Roasted by the Austrian Alpine sun, my face burned like a fire that nothing could put out or alleviate. The pain was intense and stopped me from falling asleep. Like a martyr, I decided upon a—as I thought—drastic treatment with PJ. The quality of the burn changed for a little while, but it didn't get any worse. Shortly thereafter, I fell asleep. I woke up three hours later—without any pain! And, except for a light brown-toned redness, nothing more could be seen of the sunburn. I didn't have any pain nor did any skin peel off my face afterward.

Put a few drops of PJ on your skin, rub it in a little, and then let it soak in. That's all there is to do! The Tachyonized active ingredients do the rest of the work. They help the body directly at the point of the disturbance, bind and eliminate the acids and toxins, promote the circulation, turn up the resistance, and organize everything necessary for healing.

Here is a secret tip for connoisseurs: Put 15 to 20 drops of PJ into your bath water. Even absorption through the entire body surface leads to deep muscle relaxation with a simultaneous energizing of the entire organism. This is a bath in cosmic waters!

PJ can lead to an intense reddening of sensitive skin. This is a desired effect, which may also occur more frequently if there is intensely hyperacidified tissue. This circulation-promoting effect, which is quite clearly visible to others because of its shine, should be taken into consideration before applying PJ to your face. In cases of an intolerance of arnica or niacin, first test the effect of PJ on a small area of the skin.

Components dissolved in oil separate from the substances dissolved in alcohol when the mixture remains unused for a longer period of time. You should therefore always shake it well before application to have the entire action spectrum available.

Tachyonized Ultra Freeze

In the truest sense of the word, this is the "coolest" product from the tachyon workshop. Tachyonized Ultra-Freeze (UF) is composed in such a way that it can quickly and deeply penetrate painful and inflamed tissue. Here it develops a cooling and balancing effect, above all for the muscles and tissue. The pain-relieving effect already begins after just a few minutes.

Ingredients: Menthol (7.25 percent), arnica, aloe vera, wintergreen, rosemary, lavender, broom, and others.

Application

All injuries connected with heated swelling like sprains, bruises, insect bites, and inflammations in the joints are the target for Tachyonized

Ultra-Freeze. The same also applies to heavy and hotly swollen legs and feet, as well as varicose veins and other vein disorders. Use for a tense and congested neck. Applied to the base of the skull and shoulder/neck musculature, it helps increase the circulation to a normal level and rebalance the energy flow between the chest and the head. Headaches (which are frequently involved in this syndrome) disappear and the ability to concentrate increases again.

Because of this quality, Ultra-Freeze has become an integral component of many sport bags; the work bags of physicians, healing practitioners, home nurses, massage therapists, and physiotherapists; the handbags of salespeople and secretaries; the briefcases of managers and public officials; and the glove compartments of long-haul truck drivers and field staff.

A special area of application for Tachyonized Ultra-Freeze are colds with intense formation of mucous and inflammation of the respiratory tract. The Tachyonized aromatics of menthol, rosemary, and lavender ease the coughing irritation and help the mucous membrane free itself of attached mucous. Simply apply to the chest and back for this purpose. For stubborn congestion, also dab a little at the opening of the nose and inhale deeply. For headaches, depending on where it hurts, massage UF into the temples and forehead, neck, or into the region of the head's highest point.

Absolutely avoid any contact with the eyes!

The combination of Tachyonized Ultra-Freeze followed by Panther Juice and/or Tachyonized Massage Oil potentiates the balancing effect produced by the individual remedies.

Tachyonized Ultra-Balance Massage Oil

Tachyonized Ultra-Balance (UB) Massage Oil is an indispensable remedy in many massage practices around the whole and valued skin-care oil that envelops the body in an aura of tachyon all day.

Ingredients: Oil of sweet almonds, octylpalmate of coconut oil, kukui-nut oil (Hawaiian remedy), canola oil, Vitamin E

Application
UB massage oil is an outstanding instrument for all massage therapists and bodyworkers: For hours, the soothing treatment lingers on

for the clients or patients, letting them look forward to their next appointment. Intensely moving massage work or therapy forms that work in the deep connective tissue, moving a great deal within the client, can be more easily and quickly integrated in a skin that is enveloped in tachyons.

The second essential aspect that makes the use of Tachyonized massage oil so popular is the way it protects the person giving the treatment against dissonant energies, particularly when working with the ill. The tachyon layer between the body and the hands immediately transforms chaotic frequency patterns into those that are experienced as well-ordered and pleasant for both parties to the same degree. On the one hand, this demands the trust of the client, which very much accelerates the dissolution of tensions; on the other hand, this makes the work more fun and results in less exhaustion, even on days of intensive treatments. In addition to the necessary technical quality of the work, these are all preconditions for a successful, flourishing practice.

Report from This Type of Practice

A masseur had run out of his Tachyonized Massage Oil, so he used another kind from his previous supplies to give the treatments. All(!) of the clients who he had already treated a number of times with the Tachyonized Massage Oil then asked him what was different about his treatment on that day. They weren't particularly dissatisfied but, it was somehow different. He hadn't anticipated such a response from his patients. Now he doesn't let the Tachyonized oil that flows through his hands run out.

As mentioned at the beginning, UB Massage Oil not only plays a big role for professional use, but also as a personal body oil for daily skin care, as a loving present for your partner, and for the care and massage of infants, etc.

The oil is easy to wash out of clothing and sheets. Instead of a greasy shine, it leaves a silky soft shimmer on the skin.

Its composition of high-quality oils has prompted some users to fill their daily requirement for unsaturated fatty acids with the UB Massage Oil. These fatty acids are required by the body to build supple and well-functioning cell membranes, form a series of important hormones (such as the sexual hormones), maintain the brain functions, and keep many other vital bodily systems functioning.

Through the tachyon-antenna effect of the above-mentioned fatty acids, they bring the harmonizing potential into the entire fat metabolism. I personally mix Tachyonized UB Massage Oil in with my salad-oil blend, consisting of various cold-pressed organic edible oils. This improves the quality of these oils, strengthens the SOEFs in the salad, and, consequently all the SOEFs in the body that monitor and control the metabolism of the fatty acids.

Please observe the following information: The extensive use of Tachyonized Ultra-Balance Massage Oil can lead to *detoxification*, which may be experienced as unpleasant, in people who have had no contact with tachyon up to now. It is advisable to start by using a 1:1 mixture with the accustomed massage oil or only use the UB massage oil in selected, limited areas. After three to four applications, there is usually no further appreciable detoxification to be reckoned with.

Since there is nothing added to the pure oils, you can mix aroma oils of your choice in with them.

Tachyonized Ultra-Herb Massage Oil

Selected Tachyonized herbal extracts give this massage oil additional therapeutic benefits and a wonderful fragrance.
Ingredients: Almond oil, rosemary, lavender, broom, peppermint, eucalyptus oil, kukui-nut oil, Vitamin E, Oleth-2

Application
In addition to the possibilities for use described under UB Massage Oil, the warming, blood-flow-stimulating effect of Ultra-Herb is greatly appreciated for sports massage in particular.

Tachyonized Ultra-Balance Massage Cream

This water-soluble, non-greasy massage cream is easily applicable like a skin-care lotion that is absorbed well by the skin. Because of the hypoallergenic effect, the UB massage cream can also be used for especially sensitive skin.
Ingredients: Tachyonized water, octylpalmate of coconut oil, arnica extract, aloe vera, Vitamin E, and others

Application

Tachyonized UB massage cream is the remedy of choice for massaging the face, hands, and feet. The SOEFs' energizing effect remains until the cream is washed off. This extends the therapy effect, which is found to be particularly pleasant after foot reflex-zone work, for example. As a daily skin-care cream, it envelops the body in a complete, loving tachyon embrace, therefore making it possible for the skin to fulfill its tasks on all levels (exchange of heat and substances, exchange of energy through acupuncture points, elastic definition and adaptation, sensation, etc.). It feels good to be inside this kind of skin.

The UB Massage Cream is recommended and valued in particular for pregnant women since it can prevent tearing of the tissue (stria). It also keeps the skin on the belly and perineum soft and elastic. Routinely massaging the belly in which the new human being grows can also have a medicinal benefit for everyone involved, especially the father. It can become a ritual of loving care and deep connection. After the birth, the same ritual helps the highly strained belly make a balance recovery.

I have also received wonderful feedback from gardeners and construction workers whose hands were no longer as dried out, chapped, and callused once they began using the Tachyonized UB Massage Cream.

Tip: You can occasionally pamper the people you love by applying the UB Massage Cream to their feet as an ancient sign of recognition and appreciation.

Tachyonized Passion Dew

Tachyonized Passion Dew (PD) is a special kind of lubricant. As opposed to most lubricants available for sale, it doesn't suppress the activities of the mucous membranes. Instead, it promotes the balancing production of the body's own love juice, as well as increasing the sensitiveness of the entire affected tissue.

The artfully composed mixture of components, which includes oat extract, gives PD a silky soft consistency and makes it water-soluble. It is therefore also tolerated well by condoms.

Background Knowledge: Sexuality and Hormones

Many traditions honor the body with its needs and possibilities and do not estrange spirituality and sexuality from each other through a deep abyss of taboos and concepts. These traditions have passed down to us practices for increasing and refining the flow of sexual energy. It can then be used for personal development, as well as for a loving and mature relationship with love partners and the entire world. The thousand-year-old tradition of Tantra, for example, teaches the possibilities of experiencing the unity of All That Is through full development of sexual energy. This includes the ability to make love in a loving embrace with a partner who also has achieved the same level of development.

An essential component of these traditional techniques is the contrary dynamics of masculine and feminine desire, caused by completely different hormonal regulation. While testosterone makes quick and strong stimulation possible for the man, with a climax that can be reached just as quickly, the estrogens in the woman direct a much slower increase of physical desire within her. This includes the potential for experiencing a climax that extends over a longer period of time. Only when the man learns to adapt to this dynamic, which means holding back his fire until the woman has developed the corresponding intensity, can the desired, delightful merging occur and the energies become unified.

The unifying effect of the tachyons brings valuable and desire-filled support at precisely this point. Not only men experienced in Tantra praise this support in the highest tones, but also those intensely interested in the aspect of sharing a loving embrace.

Even if this is now considered a "hot" tip in Tantric circles, the idea for the Tachyonized Passion Dew was based on requests by women in menopause. During this time, the readjustment of the entire hormonal balance, mainly through the decrease in estrogen production, can lead to the mucous membranes drying out. This can make loving union painful or even impossible.

PD now is also finding an important area of application in obstetrics. A friend of mine, who is a midwife and trainer for tachyon practitioners, told me of Passion Dew's supportive effect for the opening phase of the cervix and the elasticity of the birth canal. Through her work with Tachyonized tools and the abilities that the Quality of One process has revealed in her, she has been able to help many women in labor have a balanced and relatively short birth. This also includes my wife and the birth of our son Jona.

Tachyonized Hair Tonic

A very special mixture of specially selected, powerful nutrients in combination with tachyon makes this hair tonic a potent remedy for all forms of hair loss. It penetrates into the follicles and nourishes the hair from the root. This makes it possible to stop certain forms of hair loss within a period of 6 to 8 weeks, including many cases of patients undergoing chemotherapy who have been able to keep their hair because of tachyon. Above all, men in the best years have been able to prevent the thinning of their hair through the routine application of Tachyonized hair tonic.

From the Practice

A friend and practitioner trainer for whom time has begun to leave its mark of sparse hair on his noble head, exposing the regions of highest points on his head almost completely, demonstrates the effectiveness of the hair tonic to his course participants. He bends his head down in front of each of them and invites them to run their hands over the thick, delicate down that has formed on exactly these points during the months of using the Tachyonized Hair Tonic on a regular basis. Incidentally, he swears by all that's holy that only scientific curiosity—and not vanity, as people have gossiped—sponsored this personal experiment.

The effectiveness of the Tachyonized Hair Tonic is not limited to cases where the ravages of time have already begun to show. Treatments on a regular basis every few weeks also maintain healthy hair and counteract the manifestations of age such as graying and the loss of fullness and elasticity. The Tachyonized molecules are integrated into the hair and concentrated in it, transforming it into a gentle antenna for tachyon. This continuously supplies the SOEFs of the head with organizing energy.

Sprayed on before meditation and rubbed in lightly, the tonic activates the uppermost energy center. This facilitates the natural connection of this center to its higher levels. It creates a clear head, makes it easier to concentrate or contemplate, and frees us from halos that are too tight.

Further suggestions for applications are on long train, plane, and car trips; computer work; tension headaches; balancing dry or oily hair; and pampering your loved ones with an extraordinary scalp massage.

Please remember: Hair loss can also indicate disturbances in your metabolism that may be more severe than the aging process. In many cases, disturbed intestines with inadequate digestive efficiency play an important role. Taking mineral preparations alone can hardly provide significant help here. In such cases, ask for assistance from qualified physicians or healing practitioners.

Tachyonized
Skin-Care Products

The outstanding quality of Tachyonized skin-care products is the rejuvenating and invigorating effect even on skin that life has already marked with maturity and experience. Used on a regular basis, the exterior appearance will once again increasingly reflect the timeless beauty of the inner being.

There are four different products for various skin types and needs. What they all have in common is the excellent quality of the raw materials, approximating food quality and free of mineral oils and animal products. Absolutely no animal testing of any type is connected with the manufacture of these extraordinary skin-care products.

Tachyonized
Ultra Pure Vitamin A Anti-Wrinkle Cream

Vitamin A has been recognized as an essential active substance for the regeneration of wrinkles. In the process, the regulating effect on the production of sebum and the water balance plays a decisive role. The Tachyonized UA-1 Cream becomes active at precisely this point. It helps keep the skin smooth and elastic, balance the sebum production, and stimulate quick regeneration of the skin. An application of one thin layer provides the skin with balancing Tachyon Energy throughout the entire day. SOEFs that have been strengthened in this manner are also capable of more easily balancing external disruptive influences and thereby even maintain the protective function of the skin when it is intensely stressed.

Tachyonized Ultra Pure Vitamin A Cream can also be used as the basis of make-up.

Tachyonized
Ultra Pure Vitamin E Moisture Cream

This cream has been developed to more extensively support the protective function of the skin. On the one hand, it does this with moisture-regulating, pure active plant substances that develop their rejuvenating effects deep within the tissue; on the other hand, Vitamin E with its antioxidant effect plays a significant role in deactivating the free radicals. Free radicals are highly aggressive chemical compounds that are produced mainly during the processing of oxygen in the skin, as well as through the effect of UV rays from the sun. If such free radicals are not caught in time, they set their surroundings on fire. This plunges the affected cells and tissue into chaos and increases the tendency for cancer to be formed. On many levels at the same time, the use of UE-1 Cream therefore offers a potent aid for the skin so that it can even continue to do its task under difficult circumstances.

Background Knowledge: Skin Function

An essential function of the skin is the elimination of toxins, which is why it is called the "third kidney" in the tradition of natural healing. A large group of elimination therapies uses the path through the skin and achieves good results with it, even for chronic illnesses that are difficult to access.

The reversed path is taken by large sectors of the cosmetic industry. They mainly focus their attention upon fighting the visible consequences of toxin elimination, primarily in the area of the throat and face, by preventing the passage of the toxins with its products. The simplest method for doing this is gluing the pores of the skin shut with fat-containing substances. Although this approach creates a feeling of elasticity and simulates the idea of protection and skin care, the flip side is its lid-like effect in hermetically sealing off the skin. As a result, the organism looks for another exit or stores the toxins in deeper layers of the tissue. By using any of the Tachyonized skin remedies, an intensified detoxification may occur: the formation of pimples or impure skin for a short time as a result of optimizing the skin functions and opening the paths of elimination. Welcome your skin's regained ability to cleanse itself. In no case should you suppress this process.

Both of the following skin-care products can be used if your skin has strong reactions.

Tachyonized Retinyl Gel

Tachyonized Retinyl Gel is quickly absorbed by the skin and supports the regulation of moisture. It is composed in such as way that it is even tolerated well by very sensitive skin.

Tach-O-Vera Gel

Throughout the world, the extract of the aloe vera plant is considered one of the most significant natural healing and skin-care remedies. Tach-O-Vera is 98.8 % pure aloe vera, which this superlative healing remedy makes available in almost its original form. With the additional Tachyonization, it can be used for almost all disorders of the skin including sunburn, rash, itching, blood effusion, bruises, slight burns, insect bites and stings, acne, furuncles, cracked skin, sensitive and inflamed nipples when breastfeeding, after shaving, and many other applications. Tach-O-Vera should always be included in every first-aid kit and vacation suitcase.

Products for Inner Use

A new fascinating chapter of healing and development begins when we absorb and integrate Tachyonized minerals, vitamins, herbs, and other nutrients in our bodies! We are now capable of guiding tachyon antennas directly into specific organs and tissue. Hhere they can continuously energize the corresponding SOEFs on the spot and therefore produce the desired healing and/or balancing effect. The organs themselves will then gradually become antennas for the rejuvenating, harmonizing energy of the tachyons.

In comparison to the non-Tachyonized raw materials, the products presented in the following section have a much higher biological effectiveness, which means that lesser amounts of them need to be taken. I urgently recommend that people who do test processes with the pendulum, divining rod, single-handed divining rod, or kinesiological muscles tests take the section on *Measurability of Tachyon Energy* (page 123) to heart and mind!

As explained in the theoretical background of this book, an overdose of Tachyon Energy is not possible. However, in order to have a *detoxification* that is graceful and peaceful for the entire organism, please adhere to the dosage recommendations resulting from the wealth of experiences by thousands of users. The slow path often leads more quickly to the goal.

Among the Tachyonized products for inner use are: Tachyonized Water, Silica Gel, and Blue-Green Algae.

Tachyonized Silica Gel—TSG (Silicic Acid)

Silicic acid (silica, colloidal quartz crystal) is the most frequently occurring material in the crust of the earth. Its task in all life forms on this planet is associated with the formation and maintenance of stability and form. We find it especially concentrated in the human body wherever firmness (bones, cartilage, ligaments), elasticity (skin, mucous membranes, organ membranes), and form (connective tissue, healing of wounds) are required.

The silicic acid used for the Tachyonization process is highest quality and additionally dissolved in Tachyonized Water. This makes it into a powerful tool. For four years, it was only possible to obtain this product through professional healing practitioners. It was first released for public sale in 1996.

For the following reasons, the dosage of **two times 1-2 drops daily** must absolutely be adhered to:

The Tachyonized silicic-acid molecules are integrated into the denser and correspondingly slowest structures of our body. Since little metabolism takes place here, an accumulation of these highly effective tachyon antennas occurs. However, we find the most aggressive toxins that the body could not eliminate in particular here in these layers of tissue. They are deposited in a type of intermediate storage. The tachyons strengthen the charge of the SOEFs, which then immediately begin with cleaning up and eliminating these toxins. According to the rule of thumb: "The stronger the tachyon field, the more intensive the healing reactions and the resulting detoxification," when the dosage is too high the Tachyonized Silica Gel (TSG) can lead to detoxification reactions that may be experienced as unpleasant. This process continues until the corresponding toxin deposit (focus) has been disposed of, which can then hardly be influenced by reducing the dosage.

On the other hand, the gradual depositing of Tachyonized silicic acid leads to the entire body becoming increasingly capable of attracting Tachyon Energy on its own. This leads to a constant increase of its vibrational rate. In addition, clinical observations suggest that with "...**Tachyonized Silica Gel we have the remedy of choice available against osteoporosis!**" (Dr. Gabriel Cousens).

From the Practice

After a severe accident, the patient of a physician friend of mine was laying on the operating table. It was necessary to saw through the bone of the upper arm. This didn't succeed at first since the bone saw was too dull for the task. The surgeon angrily demanded a new saw, but the result remained the same: the saw only lightly scratched the bone. Not until someone brought a bone saw that was used for experimental surgery on pigs was it possible to carry out the operation. The radiological clarification of this phenomenon showed no indication whatsoever of pathological changes in the bones of this patient. The surgeons were puzzled. What they didn't know was that this man had taken two times 2 drops of Tachyonized Silicia Gel on a regular basis for two years. It had allowed the crystalline structure of his bones to grow so optimally that nothing could be accomplished with a saw calibrated to the hardness of a "normal" human bone. This is a wonderful example of how an optimally balanced form also leads to an equally optimal function—in the case of a bone, to a great deal of hardness at "normal" mass.

When we know about the detoxifying effect of Tachyonized silicic acid, primarily in the area of deep bodily structures, it becomes even clearer why the standard dosage must be observed (see *Detoxification,* page 120). Physicians and healing practitioners who have special remedies for supporting detoxification reactions available to them and for whom the healing aspect stands in the foreground, also use Tachyonized Silica Gel in higher dosages for all serious forms of illness that accompany the degeneration and loss of functioning tissue. The main areas of use includes the healing of wounds for acute injuries, broken bones, torn ligaments, operations, as well as all forms of spinal diseases (rachiopathy), prevention of osteoporosis, and all system diseases like the various forms of rheumatism, cancer, multiple sclerosis, degenerative illnesses, and allergies.

The growth-optimizing effect of TSG makes its ingestion by pregnant women, infants, children, and young people equally appropriate. The recommended dosage for children is the same as for adults since additional silicic acid is required for building the body. Moreover, no significant detoxification through deposited long-term toxins will occur.

All in all, TSG is meant to be a healing remedy for gradually building a strong, healthy basis to transform our physical body into a super conductor for the resistance-free flow of larger amounts of universal life energy. This effect develops through the constant ingestion of low doses over a time period of several years: a carefree kind of aging that's really worthwhile!

Similar results have been reported for the use of TSG in animals. In addition to race horses and sick cows, the regular users also include many dogs and cats. Since they usually have a well-maintained connection to the source, the use of Tachyon Energy usually leads very generally to astonishingly fast healing successes.

From the Animal Practice
A completely emaciated rabbit was brought to the consulting room of a veterinarian who had only recently come into contact with Tachyonized products. This rabbit had eaten nothing for several days. It rejected all fresh foods and only gnawed at the plaster on the walls and nibbled at the wallpaper. The veterinarian suddenly, and because it was the only Tachyonized tool in her hands, had the idea of giving her little patient one drop of TSG and nothing else. The phone rang 30 minutes later and a happy rabbit-owner reported that the rabbit was now consuming all the vegetables in the house.

Inspired by this story, a similar phenomenon was reported for the dog of a course participant in Cologne, Germany. After one administration of TSG, the dog began eating like a wolf, which means it got its appetite back.

A woman from Bielefeld, Germany called me to ask about application possibilities for treating her sick horse with Tachyon Energy. When the conversation came to TSG, she enthusiastically told me that this product was already being used in her household, but by her husband. After 30 years as a blacksmith, he had been unable to work for the past five years because of serious back pain. According to the motto of: "what's good for my horse won't hurt me!" he took two drops of TSG twice daily. After one week, his complaints had disappeared!

Tachyonized Water

This preparation is a highly purified, distilled water that has been Tachyonized. (I will give more details about the recommended intended purpose at a later point.) The emphasis of its use is a manner of application that is customary and highly successful.

Background Knowledge: Water

The elementary meaning of water in biological systems has been researched and documented in a variety of ways. We are composed up to 75 percent of this substance and most analogies of liveliness and energy are related to this element. I will emphasize one aspect of the research here that, in my opinion, has not received the attention it deserves up to now because of a lack of a model. Integrated in our concept of the SOEFs and the energetic continuum, the following perceptions permit an essential insight into the explosiveness of the topic of "living water."

Water consists of one oxygen atom, which is connected to two hydrogen atoms. Supplying coherent energy in the form of highly organized SOEFs from cosmic radiation (in the clouds), earth rays (in ground water), and vortexes in natural streams strengthens the SOEFs of the water, which increases the tension of the connective angle between the two hydrogen atoms. Similar to a battery, the water molecule can also directly store and transport life energy. A corresponding charge of the SOEFs, and therefore the molecule, is absolutely necessary to support or even merely activate most of the enzyme reactions in the metabolism of a human being. This is a key aspect for the effectiveness of water in any human biological system.

Because of incoherent technical frequencies like iron pipes, chemical processing, pollution, and electrosmog, the highly complex, living SOEFs are discharged. As a result, they cannot produce tension in the water. This has effects extending beyond the erroneous and incomplete reactions in the metabolism. In addition, this undercharged water—similar to *electrosmog*—deprives our own SOEF's organizing energy by recharging itself at the cost of these coherent fields. So we lose life energy through the absorption of discharged water in our body, as well as through external contact when showering and, above all, when bathing.

The measurement for the charge of the SOEFs, the liveliness of the water, is called the bioenergetic potential. The following values have been determined:

70-120 percent for tap water from Los Angeles

200-300 percent for recognized mineral waters.

20,000 percent for water that has been maximally charged in the tachyon field (see Silica Disk)

1,558,000 percent for Tachyonized water.

These values more or less express the ability of water, by means of the highly energetic SOEFs and their corresponding molecular structure, to convey energy in order to support the biological processes in a living being.

Considering Tachyonized water's immensely high level of activity—which is about 5,000 times more active than the most potent medicinal water on this planet—it's clear that the recommended amount to be taken in America (which naturally applies everywhere else as well) should not exceed **three times 5-15 drops per day**.

It should be applied directly under the tongue, but avoid touching the dropper with your mouth. Hold the water in your mouth for about one minute. According to experience, this amount is enough to balance the entire energy field for most people and shouldn't result in any unpleasant *detoxification reactions*.

The fantastic results for the entire metabolism and energy exchange are immediately comprehensible with our model. At every point in the body reached by the Tachyonized water molecules, a charging of the corresponding SOEFs occurs immediately. This optimizes the associated metabolism. Such a process takes place in every(!) cell, in each step of the metabolism in our body—from the innermost brain cell to the outermost, active skin cell. Along the path of this water through the organism, which lasts about 20 minutes, everything is cleansed, organized, and stimulated.

The result is an increase of the entire body's energy level, an improvement in endurance, and a comprehensive balancing and energizing of the entire subtle control field (SOEFs). As a continuous antenna for tachyons, the Tachyonized water molecules never lose their potency for conveying order. This also applies when they leave our bodies, whether in the municipal sewage plant, in the river, in the rain, on the fields and in the plants, in the fish organism, in the stomach of the fisherman, or wherever else they may go. They impart the highest order according to the cosmic blueprint wherever they are.

The Kirlian photos shown here once again impressively document the energizing and simultaneously balancing effect of Tachyonized Water on the entire energy system of a human being, as depicted in the aura of the hands. The upper photos show the condition before 10 drops of Tachyonized Water were taken; the pictures with the compact and harmoniously radiating energy corona portray the state ten minutes after taking it. In addition, the test subject had a vortex pendant, the effect of which will be extensively described in a later chapter, hung around his neck. (I was allowed to use these pictures with the friendly permission of Dr. Hansen.)

Kirlian Photos
—With and without Tachyon energy—

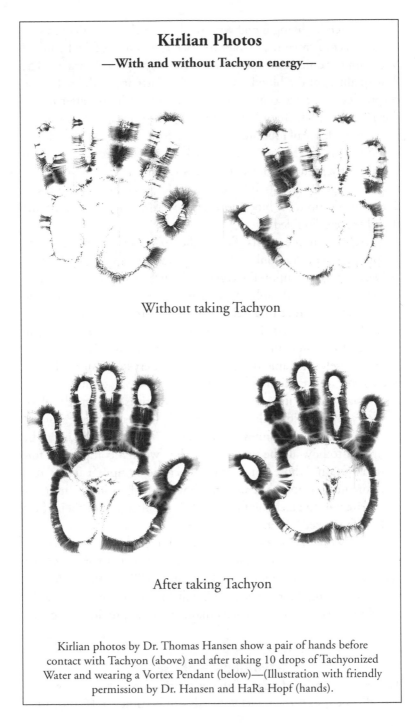

Without taking Tachyon

After taking Tachyon

Kirlian photos by Dr. Thomas Hansen show a pair of hands before contact with Tachyon (above) and after taking 10 drops of Tachyonized Water and wearing a Vortex Pendant (below)—(Illustration with friendly permission by Dr. Hansen and HaRa Hopf (hands).

Research on living blood with the help of the dark-field microscope has confirmed the extraordinary effectiveness of Tachyonized Water for the quick normalization of even high-grade disorders. The flow qualities of the blood, as well as the elasticity of the red blood corpuscles, improve so much that even a few minutes after taking the 10 drops of Tachyonized Water, the examined patients showed no more evidence of rouleaux formation. Rouleaux formation means blood corpuscles that are stuck together and clumped, which signifies a clearly reduced ability to transport oxygen and indicates the risk of clogged vessels (stroke, cardiac infarction, circulatory disorders). In addition, the blood corpuscles were documented as having their life span doubled.

Attention homeopaths, flower therapists, crystal healers, and people practicing radionics: All subtle frequencies or information patterns imprinted upon the carrier medium of water stick because of their gravitational pull. As a result, these can be transferred to living beings in order to develop their effects there. In the tachyon field, these frequencies that are foreign to the water are once again dissolved from their anchoring and the desired effect is lost as a result. Precisely the same thing happens in a crystal. All of the frequencies or information patterns that do not belong to the nature of this crystal (outside influences, programs, imprints, etc.) are dissolved in the tachyon field. All that remains is what the SOEFs of the crystal or the water manifests as its core information. This can be compared to how all the programs are lost when a computer is formatted and only those remain that affect the computer itself. It is therefore not possible to charge the above-described subtle information bearers in the tachyon field or the intensification of their effect with Tachyonized Water.

If you work with the above-mentioned therapies, you can achieve an intensification of their effects by urging your patients to always take the appropriate amount of Tachyonized Water 10 to 15 minutes before using their remedy. This will optimally prepare the energy field to respond in a balanced manner to the provided information.

Possibilities of Use

The recommended dosage of the water that has been highly purified, distilled, and then Tachyonized is three times 5-15 drops per day on a regular basis. This will gently and quickly guide your entire organism into an increasingly balanced condition, which means more energy, endurance, health, and well-being. This dose is increased for detoxification treatments or when a cold or flu is on the way. In the latter case, a little glass of the "clear stuff" can strengthen the immune system so much that it deals with the health disorder without developing any external symptoms of it. However, it is usually better to not increase the recommended dosage in the case of illness but shorten the time between taking doses of it to five to ten times 10 drops a day, for example.

Dark-Field Study on Human Blood

Sample 1
Before taking
Tachyonized Water

Sample 2
15 min. after taking 10
drops of Tachyonized Water

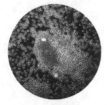

Control photos

Both of these photos were
prepared directly after the
samples were taken. The
extreme clumping of the red
blood cells in the left sample
has dissolved completely in
sample 2.

Detail 1

Directly after the samples
were taken. Observe the
structure of the cell surface as
an indication of the liveliness
and suppleness of the red
blood corpuscles (RBC).

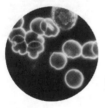

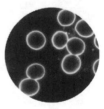

Detail 2

4 hours after the sample was
taken. All of the RBC on the
left are excessively aged and
malfunctioning, while the
cells treated with Tachyon still
show themselves to be
completely functional.

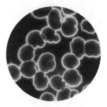

Detail 3

8 hours after the sample was
taken. All of the RBC on the
left have now been destroyed.
The cells that were balanced
by taking Tachyon are still
alive and only now beginning
to show first signs of deterioration.

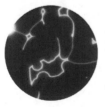

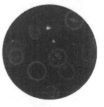

A Menstrual Problem

I know an actress from Berlin who was terribly plagued by severe complaints, which have accompanied her period every month for years, just before a performance of her one-woman cabaret. Her face was gray as ash and distorted with pain by cramps. She was angry and desperate that this had to happen right now. Like an old woman, she walked bent and complaining through the room. It was 30 minutes before the performance, so we didn't have time to do a treatment.

When she hopped onto the stage shortly thereafter and presented a magnificent show, I asked myself how she could act like that considering her symptoms. For an entire hour, she had the audience holding its breath and then clapping enthusiastically. After her performance, she came to me with a little bottle of Tachyonized Water in her hand. She had purchased it from me the day before out of pure curiosity, after I had told her about tachyons. In her troubled state, she had taken "several droppers full of it and five minutes later the nightmare was over. Not only did I have no more pain, but I was in a totally good mood and charged up like never before! Hey, that's great stuff! Phew!"

In the same way that it strengthens and balances us human beings, Tachyonized Water also helps animals. Administered directly under the tongue or mixed into the feed, it gradually increases the energy level. The animal expresses this in increased vitality, a balanced nature, and health.

Similar to how it strengthens and balances human beings and animals, Tachyonized Water also helps plants. The plants in my own household—and there are many of them—are only watered on water days (moon calendar). After the watering action, the cans are filled with water again and given a dropper full of Tachyonized Water. During the 7 to 10 days that the water remains standing, it has time to charge itself since the Tachyonized water molecules continuously attract tachyons and charge the SOEFs in the watering can. Our plants respond to this type of feeding with luxuriant green, growth, and satisfaction. They create a wonderful room climate.

In addition, silica disks or TLC Bars can naturally be used to charge the water. However, with the Tachyonized Water, tachyon antennas find their way into the plants and transform them into antennas for tachyons themselves. Cut flowers in particular are thankful for a few drops of Tachyonized Water in the vase. It also supports freshly repotted plants while they settle in new topsoil.

The highly purified, distilled, and then Tachyonized water can be used for many other purposes as well. After shaving, to pep up skin-care remedies, in room-air spray to clear and energize the SOEFs, in the bath water ... There are no limits of creativity in the different ways to use it.

Tachyonized Water is available in two different bottle sizes. The recommended approach is using the small bottles for everyday application and keeping the large bottles in the refrigerator as a supply source. Should there be clouding in Tachyonized Water, which is very rare even after storing it for a long period of time, you can always still use it to water your plants, for example.

Tachyonized Klamath Lake Algae (TKLA)

Since the end of 1997, a joint venture by David Wagner and Dr. Gabriel Cousens has made Tachyonized Blue-Green Algae from Klamath Lake in Oregon available to the public. Dr. Cousens has researched the effects of this algae as a source of food and health remedy for human beings since 1982 and come up with fascinating findings. As a result of his studies, he describes the Klamath Lake Algae (KLA): "...with an almost unlimited storage life, it is the most economical, nutritious, high-grade, ecological food on this planet." In order to clarify why Dr. Cousens would make such a statement and what this can also mean for our health and personal evolution, I will summarize some of this superlative food's benefits.

Important Preliminary Remarks

Through the process of Tachyonization, the numerous ingredients of the KLA gain fantastic additional possibilities that have an effect on our organism. When integrated into almost every cell of all the organs, glands, and tissue, they transform the body itself into an antenna for the rejuvenating, balancing, and healing energy of the tachyons. This means that of the SOEFs, with which the Tachyonized components and active ingredients of the TKLA are in contact, are continuously energized. The result has been the start of a new era in the use of Tachyon Energy for healing and development.

General Information on Algae

Algae were the first living beings on this earth (for the past approx 3.5 billion years). Through their photosynthetic accomplishments, they are responsible for about *90% of the oxygen production* on our planet. Algae are the basic building blocks of all life forms, with which they share the following characteristics:

1. With the **plant world**, the invention of chlorophyll and photosynthesis (creation of energy from sunlight)
2. With the **animal and human world**, the cell walls of protein (not cellulose, as in plants)
3. With **bacteria**, the genetic information is distributed in the entire cell (not only in the nucleus, as in plants, animals, and human beings). This makes it possible for them to adapt most quickly to any changes necessary for survival.

Tachyonized Blue-Green Algae originate in one of the last alkaline lakes in the world, Klamath Lake.

Background Knowledge about Klamath Lake

7,000 years ago, this lake was formed as a result of volcanic eruptions. Located in the Cascade Mountains at a height of 1000 meters above sea level and stretching for about 250 square kilometers, it is part of the Crater Lake National Park in Oregon. The lake has a variety of extraordinary features:

- 300 sunny days every year
- Thousands of springs with crystal-clear water
- 17 streams and rivers from the volcanic mountains
- 10-meter thick volcanic ash on its bottom (offering 60 times as much food as would be required for the simple survival of the lake)
- One of the last lakes on this planet with an alkaline environment (like the blood of human beings)
- Nature reserve, meaning hardly any civilization (people and industry: waste water, air pollution, etc.)

All in all, this is a place with highly charged SOEFs and an almost undisturbed energetic continuum! The amount of algae available for harvesting is unbelievable! Here we find enough to **provide all of humanity with 1-2 grams every day** (daily dosage of non-Tachyonized algae).

The lake's equilibrium is not disturbed in this process. The more algae that are taken out, the more grow back (because of the almost inexhaustible availability of food!) The KLA are harvested in the summer when they blossom—using fine sieves—and dried at low temperatures (which preserves the greatest amount of highly complex SOEFs, meaning liveliness, as shown by the intact enzymes and vitamins).

The Superlative Food in Detail

Proteins and Amino Acids: Our body can utilize up to 95 percent of these proteins for itself. On the other hand, animal proteins are only utilized at the rate of about 14 percent of the supplied mass. In contrast to algae and plant proteins, highly complex, animal protein structures must first be broken down with a great deal of energy exertion in order to be available for building up the body. This is like first tearing down a house that has already been built (the animal body) and having to clean all the bricks individually in order to build a new house from them (the human body). In their type, amount, and composition, the protein building blocks found in the TKLA are optimal for *immediate, energy-saving further processing* in the human body. This means they are ideal building substances.

Proteins and amino acids are required throughout the entire body, above all for building larger proteins, hormones, enzymes, and transmitting substances in the nervous system (smooth functioning of the brain: concentration, memory, intuition, etc.). We find the unbelievable amount of 300 million amino acids in one gram of TKLA.

Omega-3 fatty acids: Indispensable for the building of all cell membranes and important hormones (for example, sexual hormones) and for the undisturbed flow of cerebral activity.

Gamma linolenic acid (GLA): second-highest concentration of amino acids (after mother's milk), important for growth, hair growth, anti-inflammatory

Vitamins: TKLA contains **all** the vitamins (except Vitamin D, which is formed in the skin through solar rays) in an outstanding concentration and mixture, such as:

Beta-Carotene (17 different types!) as protection against radiation and tumors, free-radical catcher

Vitamin B-12 in the highest concentration of all previously known food (7 times higher than spirulina, which itself already has an excess of 250 percent more than an equally heavy piece of liver!). One gram of TKLA covers the entire daily need for B-12! Hooray for all vegans!

Minerals and trace elements: 92(!) minerals in a form best accessible for our bodies. Special concentrations of magnesium and iron, selenium, germanium, titan, vanadium, and many others.

2000 enzymes: Enzymes are in part highly complex substances that translate information from the more subtle areas of our energy field into the physical level. This makes possible the metabolic steps in the body, which are generally just as complex: From the digestion of the nutrients, through the acquisition and application of energy, up to the complex actions of our nervous system like thinking, remembering, and wanting. The enzyme content of foods can be equated with the amount of highly complex, energy-rich SOEFs (equated with "liveliness") that they bring into our organism. As a result of being heated to over 40 degrees centigrade (104 degrees Fahrenheit), as well as subjection to radiation and chemical clubs, the highly organized SOEFs are destroyed together with most of the enzymes. This is one more reason to support farmers who provide us with foods that have been cultivated in a way corresponding with the energetic continuum, free of herbicides and pesticides, genetic manipulation, and radioactive treatment.

Special Substances Discovered in TKLA

Phycocyanin: Is only produced in micro-algae! It stimulates the stem cells in the bone marrow to form white and red corpuscles, which means the immune efficiency and energy supply is strengthened. Because of it, there has been a dramatic improvement in the condition of children with radiation sickness around Chernobyl. Also counteracts sunburn.

Glycogen: Instant sugar in storage form, directly available without any liver activity

Rhamnose: Unique, biologically effective sugar that is responsible for the transport of important nutrients across the blood-brain barrier.

Mucopolysaccharide: Important for the building of cell membranes.

Scientifically Documented and Healing-Supportive Effects of KLA

For low blood sugar (hypoglycemia), diabetes, chronic exhaustion syndrome, anemia, tumors, hepatitis, cancer, weak immune response, virus diseases, radiation diseases, etc.

Special Effect of TKLA on Our Nervous System

In addition to all the above-mentioned components and qualities of TKLA, one spectrum of its effects will particularly interest people who want to develop their spirituality and extend their consciousness beyond their own four walls to experience unity with All That Is. This current book was created with precisely this intention, and this is the significance of applying Tachyon Energy at all. The experience of unity requires a vessel that can gracefully accept the flow of universal life energy and pass it on. On the physical level, this vessel is our nervous system. However, it is inseparably integrated and cross-linked with the totality of the body. The high concentration of neuropeptides, the basic building blocks for forming the transmission substances for nerve activity, probably makes the TKLA into the most unusual consciousness stimulant and brain tonic available today.

Research by Dr. Cousens indicates that there are special effects on the **pituitary gland, pineal gland, and hypothalamus.** These three centers regulate and coordinate the autonomous nervous system, immune system, and glandular system. They are connected to the higher spiritual centers. The Tachyonized building substances integrated into the gland tissue gradually transform the entire organism into an antenna for tachyons. This lastingly energizes the SOEFs. It makes possible a harmoniously coordinated metabolism on the executive levels of all hormone glands, of the immune troops, and the entire autonomous nervous system. In this way, the body functions increasingly in optimal balance. This also explains the following observations by people who take the blue-green algae from Klamath Lake on a regular basis:

• Increased mental alertness
• Better short-term and long-term memory
• Intensified creativity

- Heightened ability to visualize
- Improved sense of well-being and feeling of being centered
- Deepened meditation

Corresponding results have been observed in individuals with health disorders of the nervous system like depression, autism, and Alzheimer's disease. Dr. Cousens has received reports on stopping the deterioration and, in some cases, reversal of the symptoms.

Quite generally, reports are accumulating about the experiences of people who take the Tachyonized Klamath Lake algae. Since it was difficult to make a selection from them, I have stretched the scope of this book to present more of the scientific background and research on the topic of TKLA. Far from fanaticism, but with great enthusiasm, I warmly recommend this information to everyone's heart, metabolism, and, above all, nervous system. I hope that many people will get just as much benefit from taking TKLA as I personally, and many of my friends and patients, have.

Suggestions for Use

In order to experience the greatest possible success in taking the TKLA, I recommend the following:

- The best way to drink it is in the morning **on an empty stomach** or 20 minutes before lunch in some water and juice, mixed well in a shaker or blender. Because of the energy-mobilizing effect, you may have difficulty falling asleep if you take it in the evening.
- The biological effectiveness of blue-green algae is increased by the Tachyonization , which results in a **daily dosage of 1/4 to 1/2 teaspoon (0.25-0.50 grams)**. Please remember that the optimal individual dose will vary. It's best to experiment over a longer period of time with one specific amount respectively.
- For detoxification treatments, increase the dosage.
- Drink at least 1.5—2 liters (quarts) of water every day.

Note:

As already mentioned in the introduction to this section, it is not possible to overdose on this food. But be aware of intensified detoxification reactions or a hyperactivity of your body-mind system, If necessary, temporarily reduce the dosage! For many people's immune systems, the introduction of TKLA is the first opportunity for a long time to run at full speed and clean things up. Research with non-Tachyonized KLA has shown that within 20 minutes of taking the algae, the activity of the killer T-cells increases about 60 percent. This shows an enormous increase in performance for the "ground troops" of our immune system, which are responsible for cracking down on hostile bacteria nests in the body (sources of contagion). I have quite consciously chosen a military language in order to do justice to the warlike clean-up work that can be experienced here. (Also see the section on *Detoxification*.)

Because of the above-mentioned reasons, it is advisable to begin with a lesser dosage for intensely weakened and/or chronically ill adults so that the body can slowly get used to the increased quantity of energy!

In closing, here is a detail that will contribute to the much-discussed question about the price of Tachyonized materials. (Anyone who has become familiar with them and values their effects is aware of the high degree of technical expenditure for their production and who has gained enough insight into the motivation of the people making them will no longer ask this question.) The price of the daily dosage for TKLA is lower than for the conventional blue-green algae preparations! On the one hand, this has been possible through the excellent understanding between the operating companies at Klamath Lake, who reward the value of Dr. Cousens' research work for the KLA with favorable purchasing prices. On the other hand, it has benefited from the constant further development of the Tachyonization process with the lower costs resulting from improved equipment monitoring. Ultimately, the doubling of the biological activity of the TKLA on the basis of the tachyon effect makes it possible to cut the dosage in half. All of this, together with the decision to make the Tachyonized remedies available to humanity at the lowest price possible, has made this economic "wonder" possible.

Tachyonized Klamath Lake Algae is available in the 1/4-pound jar (7 months) or 3/4-ounce jar (approx. 6 weeks).

If you take 0.5 grams (two times 1/4 teaspoon of the Tachyonized Klamath Lake Algae per day, a 1/4-pound jar will last for over 7 **months!**

Tachyonized Special Products

David Wagner has created these tools in order to place potent remedies in the hands of people for their transformation. They are meant to activate and promote a powerful, graceful, and easy process.

Of the four special tools introduced here, the Tachyon Personal Cocoon and the Sun Spots are available commercially. The TLC Bar and Vortex Pendant require background knowledge, which is imparted at the corresponding seminars, for their meaningful application.

The special products are:
• Tachyon Personal Cocoon
• Vortex Pendant
• TLC Bar
• Sun Spots.

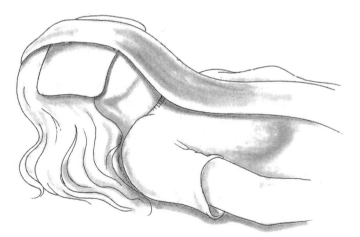

Tachyon Personal Cocoon

The Tachyon Personal Cocoon was developed by David Wagner to support and accelerate the transformation process of human beings. The effectiveness of this extraordinary instrument is based on a combination of Tachyonized tools that envelop (cocoon) the user in an intense three-dimensional tachyon field. Simultaneously, it creates a focused flow of universal life energy in which the energy centers reorient themselves back into their natural verticality. Through use on a regular basis, blockages in all levels of our being can gradually be gently dissolved. The emotional, mental, and physical bodies can be brought back into harmony with the spiritual body. This achieves harmonization and energizing on all levels of our being.

Components of the Tachyon Personal Cocoon:

The *first component* consists of two strips of a Tachyonized belt made of aero silicon fibers, like the Sleep Pad, the Life-Padd, and the Vitalizer II, which is responsible for the strong 3-D tachyon field. These two strips are joined by means of a velcro fastener and should be laid around the center axis of the body lengthwise. The result is a tachyon field that includes the spinal column, head, chest, abdomen, and pelvis—and therefore all the main energy centers as a whole.

The *second component* is the Tachyonized Eye Pillow, whose effectiveness is explained in the corresponding section of the product description.

The *third components* are the four Tachyonized Silica Disks. Two of these are inserted in the foot pocket, which is also included, in such a way that the writing—and therefore the tachyon field—points away from the feet. Each of the hands rests on one of the other two disks, whereby the tachyon field should point through the hand here.

The recommended 20 minutes a day in the Personal Cocoon have become an integral part of everyday life for many people. The immense significance of this simple measure will become clear in the following:

Background Knowledge: Regeneration and Stress

All living processes take place in rhythms or cycles. So we experience sleeping and waking rhythms, inhaling and exhaling, and our heartbeats. We know about the rhythmic alternation in the production of hormones, the building and dismantling within the body, the alternating dominance of the brain hemispheres, the cyclic activation of digestive activity, and organ functions. Based on research by the American military, various biologists, endocrinologists, gene researchers, work psychologists, and neurologists, a fundamental rhythm has been discovered, which, coded and controlled by the DNA, is common to all higher developed forms of life: the alternation between activity and regeneration. After 90 to 120 minutes of activity, an organism requires a **break lasting about 20 minutes** in order to regenerate.

During this time, for example, the transmission substances in the nerve cells, enzymes, and hormones that have been exhausted during the previous period of activity are regenerated. Metabolic wastes are eliminated and everything necessary is done in order to let the body function smoothly for the next two hours. Because of our human ability to ignore the signals that the body gives us when it is time for regeneration, we can provoke massive problems within our organism. Known as the "stress syndrome," a typical disruptive pattern develops when we exceed the activity phase at the cost of regeneration on a regular basis.

The above-mentioned scientists have described the four steps of this pattern:

First step: Concentration decreases, accompanied by yawning, tiredness, and listlessness. This is how the body shows us its desire for a phase of regeneration. The stores are empty and need to be refilled.

If a break is not taken, then the **second step:** The body must fall back on an emergency program that mobilizes its reserves and is meant to equip it for fighting or fleeing in life-threatening situations. During these phases, the stress hormones take over the command. It is often possible to continue better than before in this way since suddenly more energy is available. This gives us a sense of security—the tiredness is gone.

However, it inevitably leads to the **third step:** If no break has been taken, the body must reach even deeper into its energy pocket in order to remain a match for this continual stress. On this level, it mobilizes a nervous metabolism meant for the extreme case. Included are endorphins and neurotransmitters that make the body capable of the highest performance. This is experienced as a kick that eliminates all emotional resistance, leads a person to believe that they are "invincible" and "infinitely capable," and virtually turns someone into an addict. A workaholic is dependent upon this intoxicant of the body, which is related to the drug family of opium (morphine, heroin). However, when a person experiences this high, the result of emptied energy stores and a distorted perception of reality may be false estimations, accidents, quarrelsomeness, and so forth. The body can only maintain this phase for a short amount of time.

In the following **fourth step**, the system gradually crashes, which leads to various kinds of disturbed functions: loss of concentration, chronic tiredness, gastric ulcers, cardiovascular disorders, dizziness, accidents because of uncoordinated movement patterns, depression, loss of the sense of self-worth, etc. In order to protect themselves against this phase, many people reach for strong stimulants. These may be legal, like coffee, or illegal. In this way, they intensify the progress of the fourth phase and the certain deterioration of their productivity and health.

Applications

The solution for this very widespread impaired disorder: a 20-minute break after an activity period of 90 to 120 minutes. A break means leaning back, relaxing, and not doing anything. Only then does the genetically controlled regeneration program start up. After having made allowances for this cycle in my life over a longer period of time and, by using the Tachyon Personal Cocoon, I have been able to experience a distinct facilitation and intensification of the regeneration process.

For the normal demands of work, 20 minutes a day in the Personal Cocoon is adequate. For times of intensive concentration and work extending over several days, I recommend adhering to the 120-to-20 rhythm in order to maintain highest productivity even for longer periods of time.

I have the vision of a break room in every office and shopping center, in every factory and practice. Here the employees and bosses can spend the 20-minute breaks that the body demands in the Personal Cocoon, increasing general productivity and the overall mood. At the same time, this would avoid errors based on disturbed concentration. In these facilities, I see people being together in a balanced way, without stress and exploitation of their own resources, spending time at their work in spirit of fun and motivation.

In addition to the many users who already apply its beneficial effects for themselves, increasingly more healers and therapists are using the Personal Cocoon to support their patients/clients. Sometimes this is done before a treatment or session in order to achieve an opening for subtle and deep work. Others use it after stirring, moving work in order to facilitate quick and complete integration. However it is applied, the participants experience the use of the Tachyon Personal Cocoon as an enrichment of their work or therapy experience.

Reports on Experience

The stories of experiences that Cocoon-travelers have had are as diversified as they are numerous. The incredible spectrum of rich experiences ranges from simple pleasant relaxation to full-blown astral journeys with out-of-body experiences, from fascinating cases of healing (migraine, depression, breast cancer, etc.) to deep spiritual experiences of light, unity, and infinite happiness! To express my joy and appreciation of this excellent aid, I have selected a text depicting the experience an artist friend of mine had in the Personal Cocoon, written in verse form:

Cocoon
Immersion into stillness
Coming home to myself
Being safe and secure
In an endlessly wide, empty room
To feel myself
Like an octave vibration
In infinite space -
Even, steady, absolutely in tune
In its pure, cosmic frequency
Feeling the space of silence
In which everything resonates
Children laughing, bees humming,
Blossoms blooming so warm, so sweet
Like a sunny afternoon
In a meadow of flowers

So cool and refreshing
Like a crystal grotto
In the mountains.
(C.R.)

Important Note about the Cocoon

I advise against therapeutic work during the time in the Personal Cocoon. The large-scale balancing processes that the SOEFs want to organize should not be disturbed by anything in the outside world, even if it appears to be quite tempting to use the openness of the Cocoon-traveler for the therapist's own intentions. The use of music can also be wonderful one day, but unbearable the next time. Even within one session, the acceptance of a specific music may change a number of times. If music is to be employed, I recommend soft sounds without contours and singing, murmuring along in an even melody line.

To better understand the extensive effects of the Tachyon Personal Cocoon, I would like to once again point out the following topic areas depicted in various chapters of this book that also relate to the experiences in the Personal Cocoon: verticality, hemisphere synchronization, sunlight and gland stimulation, and detoxification.

Vortex Pendant

The Vortex Pendant is a pendant consisting of a specially cut, flawless quartz crystal and a Tachyonized cell. The model of VERTICALITY can be used in order to demonstrate its significance for human spiritual development and transformation. Every living energy system of this universe shapes, maintains, and develops its form of existence according to this universal basic pattern—with one exception: the human being! With the gift of the FREE WILL, it was possible for us human beings to create a horizontal energy system, which separates us from the source and therefore represents the starting point for many levels of disorders. Regaining the vertical energy flow is the precondition for a conscious life in unity with ourselves, our fellow human beings, nature, and All That Is. VERTICALITY is the key to a frequently prophesied Golden Age, in which the human beings recognize their place in the universe and manifest their divine nature down to the level of physical form.

Verticality—The Key to Unity

All energy systems, except for human beings, are vertically attached to the source. This is how they are integrated into the inexhaustible flow of universal life energy, which we have also called the energetic continuum. The vertical flow of energy can be portrayed through the example of a tree: Energy enters through the crown, runs along the trunk and on through the roots into the ground. In elliptical loops, a part of this energy rises from below the roots to the outside again, where it rejoins the vertical flow from the source above the crown (an apple cut lengthwise also shows this energy pattern quite wonderfully). So the tree is connected with both heaven and earth, as well as with its environment through the elliptical backward flow loops. We find this structure in all life forms as an energetic basic matrix, which keeps all things connected with everything else.

The Horizontal Energy System of the Human Being

The human energy system works horizontally, with the exception of newly born, dying, and enlightened people, because we have long been separated from the source. Many myths and theories are centered on this "expulsion from Paradise." However, it doesn't really matter whether or not we know the exact reasons. It happened—that much is clear! For our energetic structure, letting go of the source means cutting our physical, emotional, and mental bodies into pieces. This results in separation from the spiritual body. We then experience ourselves as separate from human beings, nature, God, and ourselves. So we seek security, self-worth, and love—the reconnection (Latin: religio) with the unity, the "lost paradise," in the outside world. But what we find in the outside world only reflects the state of disrupted energy fields: a mass consciousness characterized by fear, violence, and poverty.

Of the seven main energy centers (Sanskrit: chakras), only the crown and root centers function vertically, meaning open to above and below, in a horizontal energy system. The remaining five chakras are tilted 90 degrees to the horizontal. Like a ray of white light through a prism is broken into seven colors, the one consciousness reflects itself in exactly the same way in fragments, partial aspects, on its path through a horizontal system. Because of this, many problems develop. These have become so routine that we are used to juggling them like hot potatoes from one hand to the other, burning ourselves and others on them once in a while. We devote ourselves to the hope that they will cool off at some point. In a horizontally oriented energy system, there is hardly a possibility of getting rid of them once and for all so that we can use our hands for other tasks. Many great teachers and masters of humanity have developed systems along the lines of this problem. These systems are meant to cause their successors and students to recognize the hot potatoes and cool them off or let them fall. Consequently, here are the two greatest problems that we experience with a horizontal energy system:

Problem No. 1: The horizontal flow of energy only allows *giving* or *taking, transmitting* or *receiving*. Many of us have been raised to "give," but the "receiving" is usually shortchanged. This creates an imbalance within ourselves and with others. But no matter which of the two sides we are on, we always experience ourselves as separate from others.

Problem No. 2: Attention cannot be focused on more than two of the energy centers at any one time. As a result, these then determine the sector of the greater whole that becomes our conscious reality. The rest of the centers move into the shadows and influence our experiences from there. A fragmented energy field leads to fragmented consciousness that perceives the world as a place of scarcity, isolation, and danger. All the measures that we take in the desire to protect ourselves only lead deeper into isolation and separation from the source.

The Vertical Energy System

In contrast to this, all seven main centers are opened upward and downward in a vertically connected energy system. This guarantees a continuous and uninterrupted flow of the universal life energy through every chakra or level of our being. This leads to the experience of being embedded between heaven and earth, nourished and supported, and connected with All That Is. At the same time, this vertical flow of energy means the reunion of the physical, emotional, and mental bodies with the spiritual body into a totality: Everyday life and spirituality merge with each other into a common playground for our consciousness. Our bodies, nourished and guided by the energy of the inexhaustible source, blossom into their highest level of development. They manifest the following areas of experience:

- *Physical body*   =   radiant health and capacity to act
- *Emotional body*   =   unconditional love and peace
- *Mental body*   =   clarity of mind and wisdom
- *Spiritual body*   =   experience of unity with All That Is

For many people, these areas of experience represent the goal of their path. However, they are only at the beginning of a fulfilled and effective life on this planet.

The Role of the VORTEX PENDANT

With the help of the Vortex Pendant, it is now possible for us to achieve lasting verticality. Through this tool, what individuals have been able to encounter during peak experiences or deep meditation increasingly occur in our daily. We have the confluence of the essences from the lifework of three ingenious spirits to thank for the existence of this aid: 1. David Wagner with his invention of Tachyonization and understanding of verticality, who also "invented" the Vortex Pendant; 2. Marcel Vogel, a crystallogist at IBM and his epochal discoveries on the effects of crystals; 3. Drew Tousley, who with his extraordinary talent as a crystal-cutter has translated Marcel Vogel's ideas into physical form.

The result of this mutual effort is both a piece of jewelry and a tool. It creates a spiral-formed energy field (vortex) so strong that within a few hours after a person puts it on, all the horizontally tilted energy centers jump back to their natural, vertical orientation and remain there. This begins a process peaking in the completely conscious embodiment of our divinity. Such a development runs on its own dynamic, resulting from the purifying and accelerating flow of universal life energy through the energy system unified by the Vortex Pendant. Existing blockages and personality structures that do not express the essence of our being are "routed," making it possible to eliminate them. This also determines the speed and quality of restructuring our being. In order to experience this process in a graceful and effective manner, as a sort of driver's license for a vertical energy system, David Wagner has developed something else:

The Quality of One Seminar

In just three days, as *one* aspect of the training, participants are taught the conscious approach to the vertical system and the conscious reintegration into the visible and invisible energies that surround us and connect us with All That Is.

As the *second* aspect, techniques are imparted for supporting the comprehensive cleansing process (*detoxification*) that is initiated as soon as a person begins to function vertically. Old personality portions and blockages on the mental and emotional level, as well as their anchoring in the physical body, are exposed and washed up to the surface. From here, they can finally be dissolved and eliminated. The horizontal energy games of "fighting," "defending," "controlling," and "refusing" have an end put to them. Now there is space for completely new forms of nurturing and blissful togetherness with other people and all of nature.

According to the amount of stagnated energy that a person has collected during the course of his or her development, and according to his or her diligence in using the offered techniques to either get things flowing again or avoid other stagnated energies, the stabilization process of the first phase, **Level 1**, usually takes 4 to 8 months. Afterward, the system remains mostly vertical, even during difficult situations in which the person would usually fall out of balance and go back into the old, well-worn behavior patterns of fight and protection.

The next level, **Level 2**, brings a variably cut Vortex Pendant for all those who want to go further. This pendant makes possible a multiply accelerated flow of the universal life energy through the system, which has now been cleansed. The result is a frequency increase on all levels of being. This intensified flow of energy has indescribably enriched and activated many people's clairvoyant possibilities, including my own.

The teachers of the Quality of One Seminars recognize and honor the uniqueness of each human being and his or her individual path through this life. They impart no new dogmas or rigid concepts but simply provide a tool for transformation, together with recommendations for its most meaningful use. They create a space that makes it possible to experience verticality, allowing it to be gracefully integrated into the individual life path of each seminar participant. Gardeners and physicians, white-collar workers and housewives, rabbis and Christian ministers, 20-year-olds and 84-year-olds, physicists and mailmen, healers and musicians, athletes and senior citizens, men and women from a variety of backgrounds, age groups, and interests have come together in the same seminar to accept this gift for a developing humanity.

TLC Bars

TLC Bars are Tachyonized quartz-crystal squares with the most intensive balancing effect of all the Tachyonized tools. Their use requires the corresponding knowledge, which is imparted worldwide in the Tachyon Practitioner Training. Here are the interesting facts about the TLC Bars:

These quartz crystals are cultivated in highly specialized laboratories. Their little sisters play an essential role in the computer industry. The thickness and purity of these crystals is naturally unachievable for any quartz crystal that grows naturally. While the latter need about 60 million years in their nests within the earth to reach the corresponding size, while being subject to a great variety of disruptive influences, the TLC Bars grow undisturbed at the above-mentioned laboratory in 10 to 16 days. Even if the conditions for this growth have been created artificially, the results are still genuine quartz crystals of the highest quality and purity. Moreover, the explosively rising demand for these tachyon tools around the earth would lead to an intensive exploitation of natural quartz. As a friend of crystals, David Wagner could not justify something like this.

Because of the high manufacturing costs and in order to keep the price for the Tachyonized TLC Bars as low as possible, they are not offered for sale commercially. In addition, only those whose who have completed the Practitioner Training can acquire them. This means they are outside of any kind of business context.

In order to understand the fascinating effectiveness of this tool, follow me once again into the world of science—more precisely, into the world of living systems and a law that earned its discoverer the Nobel Prize.

Background Knowledge: Evolution of Living Systems

One basic characteristic of every living system is its openness. This is the core statement by the Russian scientist Ilija Prigogine, who connected the perceptions of biology with those of chaos research and consequently brought deep insights into life's secrets to light. Whether this relates to a human being, a termite mound, bacteria cultures, a company, structures of the state, or the biosphere of our earth: All developing systems are open and constantly make an effort to keep the absorption, processing, and release of energy in equilibrium. Stopping this dynamic at any point is equivalent to the beginning destruction and/or death of the corresponding system. With these perceptions, Prigogine probably would not have been able to convince his scientific colleagues to hang the Noble Prize, probably their highest distinction, around his neck. To his credit, he penetrated deep into the dynamics of this steady state. As a result,he brought to bring to light correlations that are easy for us to comprehend and could radically revolutionize our ideas of how life functions.

The burning questions were: What exactly happens with a system that falls out of its balance? What happens when it is subject to more irritations than it can process or eliminate? What happens when it eliminates more than is supplied to it? What has the life force developed with in order to withstand such crisis situations? How exactly does the game of chaos and order function?

The universal basic pattern with which every system reacts after it can no longer compensate for the imbalance is temporary deterioration of the existing order into chaos. Prigogine called this the **bifurcation point** because he discovered that deteriorated systems either organize themselves into a higher or a lower order. These are the only two paths that are open. In accordance with his background at that time as a chaos researcher, it was not possible for him to recognize a law that decided in which direction the system moved. So he called what happened there coincidence. Today, we know more: The attunement of the system to a higher order decides its fate after the point of bifurcation. In our model of the SOEFs, this means: If the superordinate SOEF is strong and fully functioning, it draws the deteriorated system into a higher order; if it is exhausted and discharged, this means further deterioration or destruction for the system. Here is a practical example to clarify these processes:

Let's again take the liver as an example of the above-described dynamic. (But remember that we could just as easily use a family, a company, the human body, an ecological system, a swarm of bees, a nation, or all of humanity as a system.)

As a living system, our liver works openly. This means it absorbs substances, processes them according to its task, and gives back the results of its work. For example, the response to an increased supply of toxins from food containing alcohol, herbicides, and pesticides must be an increased metabolic effort. Without causing disorders in the rest of the organism, the liver can put up with a certain level of these toxins. However, this is at the cost of its other capacities. Once the limit of the tolerable has been reached, the liver literally deteriorates at a moment that is called bifurcation (forking point). The organizing energy field that has been exhausted by the frequencies of the above-named source of disturbance could no longer fulfill its coordinating task, no longer maintain a smooth metabolism, and ultimately cannot even guarantee the unity of the cells on the level of natural functioning.

If the condition of the entire-body SOEF is weakened and discharged, the liver SOEF will now organize on a lower order than before the bifurcation. One example of this could be a fatty liver or, even more chaotic: cirrhosis or cancer of the liver. In the reverse case, contact with the organizing tachyon energy leads to the strengthening of the liver SOEF. The latter immediately begins to clean up. In turn, this leads to bifurcation in another direction this time, into a higher order. Even when we experience the course of the disease as a continuous process, the inner dynamic always progresses in leaps! And this is how every healing takes place—always! The path out of an illness into increasingly higher orders of health occurs through bifurcation, by way of the familiar initial worsening or healing crisis. These are scientifically explained and confirmed by Prigogine's model.

Now we understand in plain terms the role of the crisis, the deterioration of the old system into a lower order, as a precondition for the leap into a higher order of health. Just like I first have to take off old clothes before I can put on new clothes, I must first let go of the old order before I can enter into a new one. There is no way to get around this in our entire known universe of forms and frequencies.

On the basis of the extremely intensive antenna effect of the Tachyonized work crystals (TLC Bars), it is possible for the first time in the history of the healing arts to directly and quickly produce profound bifurcations. As a reminder: The bifurcation is not caused by the tachyons. It is produced through the intense activation of the tachyon field by the SOEFs with their outstanding attunement to the highest of all possible orders To guarantee that this process runs gracefully and quickly for the clients, and without any larger crises, the appropriate techniques are imparted in the *Tachyon Practitioner Training*.

During the TLC application, trained tachyon practitioners are capable of producing and accompanying the necessary bifurcation for the leap into a higher order until this higher order, such as freedom from pain, is achieved. TLC Bars are therefore only used together with the necessary knowledge for their effective application. The practical experience regarding how to handle them is given to successful graduates of practitioner training.

Sun Spots

The Sun Spots are an unusual tool with the highest level of effectiveness. Cultivated Tachyonized quartz crystals have been cut by Drew Tousley in such a way that each individual one spreads a spiral-shaped tachyon field over an area of about 30 to 40 meters. This results in the opposite effect of the *Vortex Pendant*, which concentrates the tachyon field. The Sun Spots are available in sets of four and meant to charge the SOEFs of large spaces such as entire houses. They create a room atmosphere that makes possible the best state of balance for the people who work or live there. This includes correcting the negative effects of electrosmog or harmonizing emotional movements and patterns released by the people in these rooms.

Accordingly, Sun Spots are a wonderful aid in all kinds of group rooms, treatment rooms, hospitals, healing and consultation practices, sales and negotiation rooms, and any other spaces that have intense energy demands placed on them. Moreover, they can be used in places where clarity, purity, concentration, and meditation need to be supported, such as churches, synagogues, mosques, temples, ashrams, monasteries, hermitages, etc. The best method is to place them in the four corners of the room in such a way that the fields they emit optimally overlap each other.

Because of their time-consuming manufacturing process, Sun Spots are like rare jewels in the tachyon family of products. They are currently only available at Tachyon Seminars.

Additional New Products

Just before the printing of this book, the continuous developmental process has yielded some new Tachyonized products, which are briefly introduced in the following:

Deluxe Eye Masks

A luxurious eye mask made of thickly lined cotton. It also includes earplugs that block out noise well and feel soft and comfortable. They have a tiny tachyon cell that energizes the SOEFs of the middle ear, labyrinth, inner ear, and parts of the midbrain. This synchronizes the hemispheres and harmonizes the labyrinth activities. Anyone suffering from motion sickness (ship and airplane), dizziness, and weakened orientation will appreciate this. Yet, even without these kinds of problems, the combination of the Tachyonized Deluxe Eye Mask and earplugs is the ideal companion for air or ship travel. It also facilitates a quick regeneration in the breaks during long car trips, is pleasant for the passenger, or simply helps in falling asleep afterwards. In addition, a small pouch provides space for two 30mm cells at the level of the Third Eye for those who meditate.

Small Phone-Cells

In a team development by ATT America, Germany, and Japan, these new, tiny telephone cells in various colors and forms have been created. The packages of six include two additional sets of double adhesive dots for attaching the cells to the edge of the cellular phone. Place two of them exactly across from each other on both long sides (at the level of the antenna) and two on the upper wide side; or, if possible, place them directly on the storage battery. In this way, even small and rounded cellular phones still fit into their protective coverings despite the Tachyon Cells.

The cells can also be used for correcting the negative effects of quartz watches and hearing aids, notebook computers, and the metal frames of glasses. Or they can be stuck onto mirrors and windows in the sense of Feng Shui.

TIP: First stick the double adhesive dot onto the cleaned, oil-free place of your choice. Then remove the second protective coating and place the phone cell on it using light pressure. Pressing it for a few seconds warms the adhesive and lets it stick more intensely.

Adhesive Dots for Tachyonized Glass Cells

There are now double adhesive dots for cell sizes 15mm, 24mm, and 30mm that are simple to stick onto the desired place on the body. Classified by the United States Government as hypoallergenic, the adhesive dots unite an excellent skin-tolerability with great adhesiveness. Yet, they can be removed easily and without pain—particularly in hot water—from the glass cells. They also leave no residue behind. The adhesive dots are only meant to be used once. Because of the resulting reduced adhesiveness, they should not be reused after removing them. In this way, the cells can remain in place for a number of days, although caution is advised when showering with hot water around where the cells are attached.

8MM Cells in Color

Equipped with the appropriate adhesive dots, these 8mm glass cells (usually sapphire blue) are primarily meant for application on acupuncture points. An acupuncture session's effects can be supported by continuously balancing and energizing the SOEFs of the corresponding points in the tachyon field between treatments. However, the non-professional can also easily and safely administer self-treatment according to the profound and ancient knowledge of Traditional Chinese Medicine. Numerous books on this topic List and illustrate the appropriate points. Instead of pressing, warming, or sticking needles into these points, simply attach the Tachyonized cells to them. As already mentioned, no overcharging occurs when using tachyon energy. There are also no false or dangerous points: Only the optimal balance is achieved time and again.

Another approach is to try feeling the entire surface of your external ear by applying firm pressure! Wherever you feel spots with an increased level of sensitivity, you can stick these cells onto them. Clean the skin with a bit of alcohol beforehand so that the adhesive holds well. In the section on *Happy Souls* shoe inserts, you will find information on the topic of *Reflex Zones*.

You can naturally also use these cells in the same way as the phone cells described above, which are even smaller.

New Products in Development

Tachyonized glass cells that are marked with an imprinted "T" in a triangle will soon be on the market. This measure helps differentiate Tachyonized cells from plagiarized products.

Chapter 3

More Details on Important Topics

Background Knowledge: Detoxification

All of the symptoms associated with the use of tachyons are forms of clean-up work. These are stimulated and controlled by the body's own SOEFs (self-healing). In order to understand the entire extent of such detoxification processes, which may occur during the application of Tachyonized tools, it is helpful to know what is meant by "toxins." I basically define toxins (poisons) as frequencies or forms that hinder a free, graceful, and harmonious manifestation of the perfect blueprint. There can be toxins on all levels of being:

The Physical-Material Level

Toxins from the outside are heavy metals (industrial waste and car exhaust fumes), insecticides, pesticides, phytotoxins (vegetable poisons), medications, addictive poisons (alcohol, nicotine, heroin, etc.), preservatives, dyes, and high-molecular animal proteins (meat, eggs, milk products).

Toxins from within are putrefactive and fermentation toxins from a disrupted intestinal flora (indole, skatole, etc.), as well as metabolic toxins (histamines, acid deposits, etc.) that occur during normal functioning and are deactivated in the liver and excreted without any problem in a healthy body.

The **toxic effect** here relates to the disturbance of natural processes within the body (digestion, regeneration, the ability to concentrate, alertness, etc.), up to the point of totally blocking vitally necessary metabolic steps (poisoning, chronic inflammations, rheumatism, allergies, Alzheimer's disease, cancer, etc.).

Considered again from the opposite perspective: Every disturbed function of the body is accompanied by a form that is just as disturbed. This is a result of blocked and/or weakened SOEFs insufficient translating the cosmic blueprint. All toxins disturb balanced functioning and must be transformed according to the healing process and/or eliminated! The ideal function of the body and state of optimal balance is radiant health, the ability to take action, and the expression of complete divine ecstasy in the physical form.

The symptoms of detoxification

On the physical level they are frequently manifest in the form of headaches, nausea, digestive disorders, loss of concentration, limited ability to think, skin rashes, increased sweating, body and mouth odor, flaring up of old symptoms, fever, pain, etc.

Emotional Level

Emotions are complex reaction patterns stored in the body. They are primarily managed and controlled in the midbrain. Emotional patterns have proved to be a wonderful aid in our development for supporting our survival in threatening situations. Outside of such danger, they represent a hindrance that corresponds with the effect of toxins in the physical body. The film-like mechanism that starts up when such structures are stimulated superimposes itself upon genuine feeling and the contact with our true being, thereby preventing the current solution of problems. The purest function of which our emotional body is capable is the sensation of unconditional love and all-encompassing peace. Other emotional patterns that we train ourselves in during the course of our development are more or less "toxic" deviations that, just like their "colleagues" on the physical level, are transformed and/or eliminated on the path to spiritual awakening!

The symptoms of detoxification

On the emotional level they are often manifested as excessive feelings (grief, anger, annoyance, hatred, fear, joy, etc.), insecurity, irritability, and quarrelsomeness (as a possibility of discharging emotional tension), increased projection or assigning blame to external triggers, feelings of reluctance, and depression (as signs of a pent-up, suppressed emotional charge).

Mental Level

The most powerful influence on our entire development is our FREE WILL, which is controlled by our world view and its beliefs. A belief is a crystallized structure (frequency) in our mental body that we can influence with the help of our cerebrum. This is how we program ourselves with responses to events in the course of our development (family, school, and circle of friends, etc.). According to such beliefs, we search for and process new impressions and occurrences. We consequently make our choices on our path. The toxic effect of a correspondingly disharmonious belief is apparent.

Here is a small example of this from my own "poison lab": events from my childhood, experienced with three older siblings who were intellectually tremendously superior to me gave me the idea that no one takes me seriously. Later, this belief repeatedly led me into similar hopeless battles in my attempt to be heard. Even if there was no reason in the outside world to do so, this internalized idea lured me to battles that precisely reenacted my childhood drama. This in turn led to confirmation of the pattern, and the cycle was complete! The detoxification of this belief presented me with certain tasks, the solution of which placed tools in my hands that today permit me to joyfully fulfill my calling as a teacher. I also see the role of chaos and disease reflected here: They teach us important lessons on our path of evolution and are stepping stones into increasingly higher levels of order and consciousness.

The view that we have of the world represents the sum of all beliefs and conceals within itself the deepest cause for human suffering, disease, and destruction. For many people, it equally represents the "golden calf," which is deeply buried in the unconscious like a treasure. As a result, the necessary learning on this level usually takes place very hesitantly. Most people do not achieve the highest developmental level of the mental body: wisdom and clarity.

The symptoms of detoxification

On the mental level they are frequently manifested in the form of poor orientation, confusion, illogical argumentation, no longer knowing what is "right" and "wrong," memories of childhood situations, mental carousels, etc.

Conclusion: All of these detoxification symptoms can, according to the status of personal development, take place in connection with each other. Consequently, old deposits in our intestines influence our thoughts on the theme of boundaries—and the nicotine in our cells influences our thoughts on smoking. Suppressed hatred obstructs the healing of skin rashes, and even the earliest childhood memories can maintain bladder infections and kidney disorders. The use of Tachyonized tools makes it possible to balance disrupted patterns. It opens up learning opportunities on all levels and leads to a far-reaching transformational process that includes the entire being.

No individual who has collected toxins is spared of the path through detoxification. But controlling the speed and intensity of this process lies very much within the scope of possible alternatives. I basically recommend that the use of Tachyonized materials be reduced if the detoxification process is accompanied by unpleasant or alarming symptoms. The friendly path usually leads more quickly to the desired results here. However, you should not in any case suppress or block the detoxification reactions, whatever type they may be. Make it clear to yourself that your healing, the experience of a higher order of health, is waiting for you on the other side of this process. Your own SOEFs are leading you in this direction. On the other hand, the strategy or intensity of the application should naturally be changed if the desired results fail to occur.

Measurability of Tachyon Energy

Have you already asked yourself how the existence of tachyon can be proved? How sure can you be of not falling for some dreamer's fantastic idea that may sound good but has nothing to do with reality? How can we measure the tachyon?

Right at the start: There is currently no known measuring method with which tachyon can be directly measured! It finds itself in good company here since gravitation also cannot be measured. But each of us can very easily convince ourselves that it exists because of its effects. The same applies for tachyon energy! But since the principle of measuring or being measurable still represents the path of the dominant scientific culture for bringing proof, the perceptions from quantum physics and mathematics still meet with skepticism or rejection even from the colleagues of the physicists. In order to understand why we must do without this source of evidence for tachyons, it is best to look at the instruments available to us:

1. We human beings have **our senses** for the perception of reality. On the physical level, these are attuned to certain frequency areas, within which we experience our world. For example, our eye functions in an area of the electromagnetic spectrum ranging from about 360 to 720 nm and our ears comprehend sound waves from about 16 to 20,000 hertz. In order to activate our sense of touch, a certain threshold value of pressure is required. A specific concentration of chemical stimulation is necessary in order for us to smell and taste. If occurrences lie outside the comprehension limits of our senses, we simply don't perceive them, even though they may very much influence us.

Conclusion

Tachyon has no frequency and is faster than light. Consequently, there is no direct interaction with our senses. This is why tachyon energy is neither visible, nor audible, nor tangible, nor can it be smelled or tasted. Only the regulating SOEFs affect changes that we can feel. Therefore, s the very individual, regulating transformation through the SOEFs is *always w*hat we perceive when we feel something. In this situation, the more blockages there are to clear out, the more distinctly this process can be perceived. The decisive proof for the existence of tachyon and its effect can ultimately only be provided by the very personal experience of increasingly more healing, balance, and development; by the process of transformation or however the development of a higher order is experienced.

2. With the help of **technical measuring devices**, we can tremendously expand the range of how we objectively perceive the outside and inner world. Telescopes, microscopes, spectroscopes, oscilloscopes...whatever equipment the human being has invented for comprehending the world works, like the senses for whose intensification they were built, with frequencies in specific ranges. Every expectation of measurability, the most important basis of scientific character since Descartes and Newton, is therefore only related to the frequencies within our limited perception.

Conclusion

As applies to the senses, even the finest and most sensitive measuring equipment that still functions only within the limited frequency range cannot capture the faster-than-light and no-frequency tachyon energy. Because tachyons are not subject to gravity, interaction with frequencies is not possible. The tachyon field that is emitted by a Tachyonized Silicon Disk, for example, cannot enter into an interaction with any frequency device; accordingly, it also cannot trigger any reactions that could lead to a measuring signal. Biological systems like DNA, plants, mice, fruit flies, and other beings that cannot be accused of having preconceived opinions and wishes provide the objective provability of tachyon's no-frequency effect.

The most spectacular scientific confirmation of the tachyon effect provided by ATT's products came from a study on human DNA. Test series, findings, and conclusions can be read in detail in the book by David Wagner and Dr. Gabriel Cousens—*Tachyon Energy: A New Paradigm in Holistic Healing*. Tachyon energy has therefore been proved in its practical effect, just like gravitation. And, to the same extent, the mathematical proof of its existence has also been provided by the work of quantum physicist Ernst Wall. This is described for anyone who is interested or mathematically skilled enough with the calculator to duplicate in his book *The Physics of Tachyons*.

3. A group of measuring procedures, which is also increasingly used by laypeople, is **radiesthesia**. With the pendulum, divining rod, or an angular or one-handed divining rod, the experienced person can penetrate into measurement areas that lie far beyond the range of technical devices. In my own healing-practitioner practice, for example, a one-handed divining rod has long served as an important diagnostic aid. **Kinesiological examinations** also fall into the same category. Instead of external tools, the strength or weakness of a muscle indicates the answer to yes/no questions in this method.

You should know the following, both as a user and as a client: The swing of the pendulum or divining rod is always related to the question asked by the user and not directly to the energy measured. In this sense, turning to the right and turning to the left are not physical circumstances like spin or isomerism. It is always solely the yes/no answer to the user's question.

The result of this is

that without the right question, there is no correct answer. Question and answer exist exclusively within the testing person's system of understanding.

From the Practice

A client had purchased Tachyonized Silica Gel and called me rather irritated a few days later. A well-known pendulum-expert had come up with a measuring result different than our recommended dosage of maximum 2 drops two times a day. His dosage recommendation was three times 40 drops. Since the dowser couldn't relate to the additional label of "Tachyonized ," his measurement was based on the customary silicic acid available in any drug store. His understanding alone produced the reference system for his pendulum swing and not the little bottle of TSG with its potential for the woman who wanted to use it. The expected detoxification process, triggered by his ignorance of the tachyon effect, would have presumably been quite "moving" for the woman.

This is probably the most serious criterion for trustworthy results from this type of measurement procedure: My expectations, even my unconscious expectations, determine the result. If the person using the pendulum, divining rod, or kinesiology is not completely free of any kind of personal motives, the results will be colored. It doesn't matter if this is an economic interest or a personal interest like validation, wanting to be right, exercising power, fears, just desiring the best for someone else, wishing to confirm one's world view, etc.!

My limitations and possibilities determine the quality of my testing. Not taking this background into consideration and believing that you are getting objective results with the pendulum or divining rod has already produced the strangest resulting in "measuring the tachyons." There were supposedly demons on them, if the pendulum only swung to the left; for others, if the pendulum only turned to the right then extraterrestrials have deposited information on them for the enslavement of humanity. For one person, they are useful and for another they are harmful... The common denominator of all these measurements is the projection of one's own ideas, limitations, fears, and expectations onto the Tachyonized tools, which become a clear mirror for the tester in this case. As important as it is to master these measurement techniques when using frequencies in the area of the healing arts to support the best possible course of therapy, they are useless when applied to tachyon energy.

Again, it is the practice that ultimately decides on the credibility and ability of the person using the pendulum. This simple test, carried out by the American Society for Radiesthesia, separates the capable from the incapable in a very simple and quick manner: Take five equally large pieces of paper and write one of the numbers from 1 to 5 on each of them. Mix these pieces of paper and then lay them out next to each other with the numbers facing downward. The task is to arrange the cards in the sequence from 1 to 5 without looking at them beforehand. How can someone discover highly complex correlations with the help of his art if he cannot even pass this simple test? Only trust those who can do this test 100% accurately and repeat it three times. Ask yourself: How can someone tell me something about what I don't know if he can't even tell me what I already know?

Perhaps I'll have the fun of compiling all the findings, measurements, channeling, opinions, warnings, fear, euphorias, along with observations by mediums and clairvoyants, and their consequences in an enjoyable reader with a title something like: *Superstition at the Turn of the Millennium.* Everything that I've heard up to now would be enough for the first volume.

With the help of the corresponding reference system, as depicted in the introductory chapter on the physical background of tachyon, we are capable of differentiating quite precisely between which statements are anchored in a reality connected with the entire Creation and which have their source in the fantasy workshop of a "private scholar" and also can only be understood there.

Background Knowledge: The Tachyon Market

Since the worldwide distribution of the Tachyonized tools invented by David Wagner, there are manufacturers who offer related products, which they say also work with tachyon energy or with zero-point energy. The general public's basic lack of clarity as to what tachyons and zero-point energy mean in terms of a scientific explanation allows any amount of speculation and theories, which have sponsored these types of products. In the following, I will give you a key to how you can find out yourself whether or not the recommended products deliver what they promise.

Zero-point energy is completely out of the question as an easy-to-handle medium for work. With the qualities ascribed to it by science (which you can read in the theoretical introduction at the beginning of this book), there can be no interaction of any type with the universe of frequencies and forms. For this reason, any products that claim to work with zero-point energy can be omitted here. Remember once again that you cannot grasp the whole itself (ZPE) with any **part** of the whole (frequency). No theory, no matter how brilliant it may appear, can obscure this. In the sense of science, we define **tachyons** as ZPE in particle form. Only as such can ZPE come into interaction with our universe of time and space (frequency and form). However, this occurs solely through SOEFs, which develop and maintain the forms and frequencies of our existence through their (somewhat slower than the speed-of-light) contact with the tachyons.

It is not possible for frequencies and forms to stop, catch, pass on, inform, or imprint tachyon energy because, like ZPE itself, it moves more quickly than light, possesses no frequency or spin, and is not subject to any gravitational pull. This would be the precondition for entering into an interaction with other frequencies. Consequently, this excludes all the products that work by informing materials (glass, sand, fabrics, etc.) with tachyons or ZPE by means of radionic devices, mental efforts, or any other manner. The former orgone accumulators also contributed just as little to enticing tachyons into our universe as electromagnetism in the high-vacuum field or atoms influenced in the magnetic field. The tricky task of bamboozling the universe out of the secret of its form and integrity cannot occur through using the frequency-specific tools with which we have been familiar up to now, thank God!

Whatever effects these products trigger, and some of the tested products did prove to have effects, can be sought and found in the range of frequencies. This particularly applies here: The frequency that can quickly balance something leads away from this newly gained balance just as quickly. As demonstrated at the beginning, the principles of every healing art also apply to these products. Not observing these rules can, particularly with "intense products," lead to disturbances of our natural processes, which are equivalent to our balance and our health. **Please remember that feeling something does not necessarily mean being simultaneously brought into balance.** An intense tingling, heat, constriction in the chest and solar plexus, headache, etc. are effects that say nothing about whether healing or injury is taking place. You as the user or therapist must comprehend the meaning of these manifestations and classify them within the therapeutic context.

A simple test series made it possible for David Wagner to check whether the above-mentioned products actually develop their effect with the no-frequency tachyon energy or by means of frequencies. To come straight to the point about the results: None of the numerous products that were examined in this manner was capable of passing the test, with the exception of those from ATT. The proof is simple, and anyone who is skeptical about the possible partiality of the tester can easily reproduce it with the corresponding expenditure for materials. Here's how to do it:

You will need a plant, along with a lie detector for registering the current of the plant or a Kirlian device for the photographic recording of its high-frequency aura, together with a frequency generator that has particularly high level of output. First, test the reaction of the plant to the respective product by using your diagnostic device. Some of them will already be eliminated from the selection since they are not at all capable of exercising a harmonizing, constructive effect on a living system. If there now is a measurable reaction in the energy field of the plant, expose your product to the chaotic vibrations of the frequency generator. This means you are destroying the more highly organized SOEFs of your product with the electromagnetic steam hammer, including the order contained in the information or frequencies. The next step is clear: Simply test once again whether the treated plant shows a reaction to your product. If yes, then you have a tool in front of you that shows its effect without frequencies, which means by way of tachyons. No reaction means that the previous effect had come about on the basis of frequency-specific interaction.

As David Wagner personally confirmed for me before the printing of this book, the results produced by this simple test of exclusion for all previously tested products clearly let us recognize the following: Only the products that David Wagner invented and are exclusively distributed by ATT (which can be seen in the protected logo) develop their effect by means of tachyon energy. Although all the other products are cheaper for the most part, they work, if at all, on the basis of frequencies. We didn't even have to test the so-called Japanese tachyon products in the first place since the English-language, original accompanying brochure clearly states that these are photon (frequency) products, which are only meant to improve the body's receptivity for tachyons.

I value the great service that the manufacturers and distributors of these products have accomplished in the dissemination of this completely new type of technology, tachyon technology. They have helped spread the concept. The chaos of terminology that has resulted offers us all the opportunity for greater clarity and consciousness in dealing with tachyon products and those that function on a frequency basis. Ultimately, it is up to each user of any kind of product to precisely sense whether it serves the development of increasingly more balance and harmony. It is also the responsibility of each individual to measure the reality of theories that frequently sound good in comparison to one's own experience, as well as investigating the integrity and competence of those who set them into the world.

"American" and "Other" Tachyons

On the topic of "expanded, European, Japanese, stronger, etc. tachyon products," by various suppliers—especially in the German-speaking countries of Europe—I would like to let David Wagner have a word himself. The following excerpts are from an interview of July 8, 1998 on the occasion of his seminar series in Europe. (Printed with friendly permission of Advanced Tachyon Technologies Europe).

Question: *Your description of what Tachyonization is indicates a multitude of products that are currently showing up around the world. These new products claim to be tachyon energy products. Are these people really making tachyon energy products?*

David Wagner: In order to understand what is happening, we must first bring a few things to mind. First of all, as a worldwide company we distribute our products in 55 countries—from Japan to Australia to India, the USA, Canada, Mexico, South America,

Singapore, Malaysia, to Puerto Rico—almost every part of this globe has already been touched by my Tachyonized products. The company is large. Our influence on the world, and that of our tools, is considerable. The proved results in connection with the knowledge that tachyon energy is not a frequency but rather the source of all frequencies has set a wave of perception in motion. These perceptions are in regard to consciousness, healing, and transformation. These revelations have pushed certain individuals into a battle for survival. Those individuals who use an old, frequency-oriented technology often just put a new label on it or attempt to depict these old frequency technologies as something that they simply aren't. Most people see through this unfortunate, misleading marketing game. They clearly see that these individuals are simply trying to survive through this false information. I'm not accusing them of anything. They have served the world and individual human beings for many years. But the world must continue to develop. First, tachyons were discovered, and then the process of Tachyonization. And now Tachyonized tools are in the process of revolutionizing the world of energy applications that we have known up to now.

Question: *Some people say that tachyon is just another word for magnetism.*

David Wagner: There will naturally always be people who prefer to cling to the past instead of developing themselves into the future. While they cling to it, they continue to try surviving by presenting old frequency-specific technologies, boosting them, re-marketing them and repackaging them in a way that intentionally or unintentionally misleads the public as to what these frequencies actually do. Older technologies from the 1970s and 1980s still attempt this restructuring by using magnets. Although machines containing magnets show their greatest potential within themselves, in relationship to tachyons they have long been mustered out. The simple reason for this is that every magnetized material can be demagnetized again through a magnetic source that is stronger than the original magnet.

There are also others who believe that zero-point energy can be produced with magnets. I have studied the work of an individual who built a chamber with opposing magnets, which he offered and sold to an uninformed public by claiming it was a device for restructuring materials for tachyon energy. At the beginning, he called it a Tachyonization machine. However, since the word "Tachyonization" is a trade name of Advanced Tachyon Technologies, my attorney was able to stop him from the fraudulent use of our name. Be that as it may, opposing magnetic fields have been used for hundreds of years to continuously produce the movement of machines and free energy or change and restructure materials. They have also been 100 percent successful in this restructuring: With the use of a magnetic field, a new magnet can be created but a new magnet is not a tachyon antenna.

Question: *What about ions and ionized atoms?*

David Wagner: I recently read a book that claimed tachyon energy is produced by a magnetizing device, which the authors sold. They claimed that tachyon energy splits off the ionized atoms from the molecules. The truth is that only frequencies can split something off. We should be skeptical about people who believe that tachyon energy shoots off or causes harm. Tachyon is the source of all frequencies, which are transformed into exactly the right frequency for the corresponding form through the SOEFs. It is neither negatively ionized—nor positively ionized—although both have the right to exist.

Question: *Why is the world so fixated upon renaming frequency-oriented devices to be tachyons?*

David Wagner: When people see or hear something, they try to understand it and adapt it to their perspective of how the world functions. Tachyon requires us to go one step further into a new era of understanding. Actually, when someone is prepared for it, tachyon brings meaning into the world of frequencies and therapies. This is why some people will welcome this scientific breakthrough and others in turn will attempt to keep their worlds the way they are and only call the old technologies by a new name. Energy is composed of countless combinations of frequencies—combinations of all of them from the lowest to the highest measurable frequency and beyond. Life as we know it enjoys the magnetic field of this planet. But magnets only represent a tiny spectrum of frequencies, but not the source of life.

Did you know that in the entire world there is only one small region in which frequency-oriented devices are produced under the name of Tachyon? This is in Austria, a place in Germany, and a little place in Switzerland. There is a company in Japan that distributes its products under the name of Tachyon. However, when you read its catalog, at least the English-language version, they tell the truth. They sell a photon-energy product with a specific frequency between 4 and 16 micrometers, which makes the body receptive for tachyons. So they are ultimately honest about the frequency information in their brochure, although their marketing strategy speaks of selling a tachyon-energy product. Anyone who understands science will see through these things. The problem is, and most of these companies reckon precisely with this, that you, the reader, don't know anything about science. They also calculate that you will believe all of their newly packaged marketing games with which they seduce you into buying their products. Precisely here is the benefit and the problem. The benefit is that more people now know about tachyon energy than ever before. The disadvantage is that when someone buys such a frequency tool and it doesn't fulfill all the awakened hopes, he will be disappointed and believe that tachyons apparently don't work.

Question: *What effects will all of these frequency-oriented "tachyon" products have on the world?*

David Wagner: These devices and tools, as well as the machines that are being offered, are in the process of exercising an initial negative effect on the possible service, healing, balance, and peace that can be achieved with the use of tachyons. On the basis of verbal propaganda, seminars, physicians, research reports, books, etc., people realize that our Tachyonized tools actually function. They may have experienced this themselves or loved ones or friends may tell them about the incredible effects. And then, out of the blue, someone gives a magnetic-flow resonator the new name of "Tachyon Restructuring Machine" and adds a bit of dated magnetic science to it. People who have learned to trust the integrity of the tachyon-user then believe this.

So you could buy a device in order to produce your own energy-frequency tools. You could even sell these tools and glut the market with cheap frequency-specific tools that you pass off as tachyon tools.

These products will not work better than the frequency tools with which they were produced. When you use these frequency products, you will not receive the blessings of the tachyons. Some people will observe an impact on the basis of a placebo effect. Others will feel something because of the kick that the frequencies cause. But, as in all the other frequency technologies that are one or two years old, the limitations will come to light and people will be disappointed. And so they may give up. If you then ask them about tachyons, they will say: "Oh, tachyons, that doesn't work anyway!" The individuals who distribute such products undermine their world and the possible healing and rebuilding of this planet through the use of tachyon energy. It is unfortunate that, through their decision to use what the tachyon energy has brought to the world for themselves, they are probably undermining the greatest gift of our time.

So you can understand that I see both the positive and the negative aspects of this. And I really love watching the dance of Existence. I find it important to recognize that there must always be polarities since no one could recognize the truth without these polarities. Our technology, as described in my book, is anchored in pure science, built upon research that has proved my discoveries. And the background of the information that we pass on is based upon irrefutable proof of what tachyon is and how it functions. From the DNA to the plants, from living nourishment to the human being, we are capable of proving that tachyon energy is not a frequency.

Tachyon Introduces a Change in Paradigm

Shortly before this book went to press, at the very last opportunity of sharing this information with you, a sensational breakthrough was announced regarding a method of measuring the effect of Tachyonized materials. A simple procedure, implemented by equipment that the American Government has confirmed to be effective, has made it possible to precisely document entropy in living systems—for the first time in the history of science. Entropy means the deterioration of the order of a system—or, expressed in different terms—the dying or aging of such a system. As a result, it has also become possible to record the effects of anti-entropic (slowing or reversing the entropy) processes of Tachyonized materials. This proof is provided in a scientific manner that is precise and easy to understand.

The results of this research are scheduled to be introduced to the world public before the beginning of the new millennium. As a result, it will be possible for anyone to simply and quickly examine anti-entropic methods (= healing systems, medications, technologies) for their effectiveness. Right at the start of the new millennium, this breakthrough will ring in the announced change of paradigm in holistic medicine and science. The thousand-fold positive healing and developmental experiences had by users of Tachyonized materials will achieve new levels of significance.

Chapter 4

Appendix

Examples of Applications

Pregnancy and birth: TKLA, Silica Gel, Tachyonized Water, Cocoon, Massage Oil on abdomen and back (every day from the start), Passion Dew (massage into perineum and vagina daily starting in 6th month), Vitalizer II, wristbands, joint hugs, Panther Juice, Ultra-Freeze (legs and feet), Sleep Pad, silk meditation wrap. For **lactation period**, additionally use: Tach-O-Vera for sore and sensitive nipples, neck pillow.

(School)Children: Silica Gel (2 x 1-2 drops), TKLA (2 x 1/4 tsp.), Personal Cocoon, headband, wristbands (possibly with emblem of favorite football team), silk meditation wrap, Happy Souls, pendant above thymus gland, Silica Disk on bed.

Workplace: TLKA, Life-Padd, Tachyonized Water (possibly in pump sprayer), neck pillow, Personal Cocoon, Vitalizer II, Silica Disk in fuse box or on monitor, silk scarf, Happy Souls, Ultra-Freeze.

Healing work: TKLA, Silica Gel, Tachyonized Water, Flexcell 100, Vitalizer II, wristbands, pendant on thymus gland, Silica Disks on treatment lounge, Sleep Pad under the sheet, Personal Cocoon, Happy Souls, neck pillow, Massage Oil or Cream, TLC Bars.

Meditation: TKLA, silk meditation wrap, Personal Cocoon, headband (plus cell), eye mask (De Luxe + 2 x 30mm cell), Life-Padd, Sleep Pad, Silica Gel, wristbands, cell on Third Eye, Vitalizer II.

Sports: TKLA, Tachyonized Water (10 min. before competition), Personal Cocoon, headband and wristbands, joint hugs, wraps, Vitalizer II, Happy Souls, Panther Juice, Ultra-Freeze, Massage Oil.

Travel: TKLA, silk meditation wrap, Deluxe Eye Mask, eye pillow, neck pillow, Vitalizer II, Ultra-Freeze, Sleep Pad, Tachyonized Water, Happy Souls, headband and wristbands.

Plant care: Place Silica Disks or Flexcell 100 under them and use to charge water and fertilizer, Tachyonized Water (in water, occasionally spray leaves with it), Silica Gel

Animal care: Pet-Pouch or Life-Capsule, Silica Gel, TKLA, Tachyonized Water, Flexcell 100, Life-Padd, Vitalizer II, wraps, headband around the neck.

Questions and Answers

In the following section, I respond to a selection of questions that have been frequently asked by course participants and patients/clients. I would like to summarize them here.

Question: *Can I combine tachyon with other forms of therapy?*

Answer: All forms of therapy that are capable of supporting the self-healing powers of a human being can be wonderfully combined with the use of Tachyonized materials. Above all, these include naturopathically oriented therapies like acupuncture, phytotherapy, chiropractic and osteopathy, homeopathy and flower therapy (observe information in section on "Tachyonized Water), crystal healing, and, above all, every form of spiritual healing like the laying on of hands, Reiki, prana healing, etc.

Measures that suppress and block natural processes can be obstructed in their effectiveness. I therefore urgently advise you **not to use any Tachyonized products during chemotherapy and radiation therapy**. This medicinal science, designed to destroy the SOEFs, competes against them for their constructive tachyon energy. So these methods may be impeded in their intended effect, which would cause the treating physician to increase the dosage. The use of tachyon should be limited to the intervals without this type of therapy.

The administration of psychotropic drugs while simultaneously using Tachyonized products should also be accompanied by an appropriately qualified healthcare practitioner.

At this point, I would like to once again emphasize that in the case of serious illness, or the suspicion of such, you should absolutely consult a qualified healthcare professional. No statement in this book has been made with the intention of questioning this important point!

Question: *Are bacteria and parasites, like candida and molds, strengthened by the use of tachyon?*

Answer: The spreading of bacteria and parasites requires a disturbed environment, a weakened and overwhelmed immune system, or disrupted SOEFs of the corresponding organs or sections of the body. Only under these conditions do they feel well, can settle, develop, and grow. Just like no bark beetle or fungal infestation can be found on a healthy tree, a balanced system rules out the attack of "pests" in us human beings. Incidentally, I think the term "pest" is rather shortsighted since the service of this life form represents an essential step in the recycling system of our biosphere. When we change the quality of the environment with the help of tachyon and the resulting strengthened SOEFs, the parasites experience much less enjoyment of their work. Our healthy frequencies weaken their SOEFs and vice versa. However, through tachyon they cannot become any stronger than they already were when they invaded our organism. They lose their own equilibrium and the charging of their SOEFs when the infested body recovers. Still, I would advise that the appropriate naturopathically justifiable measures be taken to support the body in dealing with fungus and bacteria.

Question: *Can I overcharge myself with tachyon energy?*

Answer: No! All reactions to the use of Tachyonized materials are simply and solely the regulating response by the blocked SOEFs. Through their contact with tachyon, they are once again enabled to carry out their task of maintaining balance within the system, now making amends for all the "errors." A great deal of tachyon means intense detoxification. Remember that the gentle path may take a bit longer, but it ultimately means reaching the goal (ultimate balance) more quickly. "Soft is stronger than hard, and perseverance leads to the goal!" is what the *I Ching*, the ancient Chinese book of prophecy, tells us.

Question: *Can I become dependent upon the Tachyonized products?*

Answer: In view of the findings of physics during the past 50 years, the possibility of there being anything like independence in our world has been reduced to zero. The quality of what we are dependent upon should therefore be the content of our questions. By way of strengthening the body's own SOEFs, the use of Tachyonized aids leads to the true satisfaction of our needs instead of the vicarious satisfaction that increasingly leads to new addictions. Addiction mechanisms are thereby not possible because only our very own needs are satisfied on all levels. This results in balancing into the state of who we truly are. In this sense, I am addicted to tachyon in the same way as I am to fresh air, organic food, loving people, intact nature, and so forth.

Question: *Do I need tachyon at all?*

Answer: There are a number of possibilities for answering this question.

1. As a quantum physicist, I would be astonished at this question and point out that tachyon is the source of all form and being in our known universe. Solely the continuous contact with inexhaustible tachyon energy through our SOEFs decides upon our "being or not being" in the game of our universe. How could I be without it?

2. As a theoretician, I can approach this question from all directions. I could gush about it and play along enthusiastically until other ideas drive me to new concepts. I could let my personal concept of life, God, and the universe battle against prevalent knowledge and act out all the possibilities that lie between the two extremes. I could indiscriminately change between the poles without letting myself be touched by an experience that may possibly mean the leap into a higher order of consciousness.

3. Disturbed SOEFs mean the same as a reduced conversion of tachyon. In many places, our environment is in a catastrophic condition in the form of air pollution and contaminated, poisoned, over-fertilized, genetically manipulated, radioactively treated "food," as well as in the form of energetically discharged water full of toxins and chaotic energies, and the hole in the ozone layer. Such an environment, to which we continue to be bound in the sense of our very existence, is out to get our SOEFs. With this consciousness, I reach for every—really every—opportunity that makes it possible for me to effectively protect myself and reverse the deterioration resulting from this deplorable state of affairs. In an intact, nourishing, unencumbered environment; in the midst of our healthy and strong tree friends; with farmers who work lovingly and eco-logically; in a world free of electros-

mog, herbicides, and pesticides; in a world without the battle for survival, for positions of power, and for energies of all types—In such an environment I would need no technical aids in order to lead a balanced, connected life in harmony with the Creation.

4. This ultimate goal of this entire book is to sensitize the reader about finding a personal answer to such questions.

The Global Vision

Since the first Tachyonized products were made available to the public in the year 1990, there has been an explosive distribution of these wonderful tools. Today, they are used in 55 countries around the globe to support the balancing and healing of human beings and Mother Earth. In addition, increasingly more companies are recognizing the potential that lies in the combination of their products with tachyon. These include firms like a large computer manufacturer in Japan who installs Tachyonized Silica Disks into its monitors as standard equipment and a German water-filter manufacturer who achieves an additional 20 percent increase in its water quality with a built-in Tachyonized Silica Disk. There are currently negotiations in progress with the Indian government for a water-processing project and many additional projects ranging from Tachyonized dental cement to Tachyonized raw materials for bathtubs, all with the basis of serving human beings and the entire planet.

As the next step of development, in order to make the best possible training and information for the meaningful use of tachyon energy available to the world, a **Tachyon International Institute for Spirituality and Science.**

The Tachyon International Institute for Spirituality and Science opened in America, parallel to the opening of such an institute in Europe, in 1999. The task of this institute is to educate highly qualified trainers who will pass on these new technologies in the following seminars:

Tachyon Practitioner Training Level 1: The meaningful use of Tachyonized products and pain management with the help of the TLC Bars (currently the strongest tachyon antennas) will be taught here. This seminar is directed toward professional practitioners of medical science and the healing arts, as well as people who have recognized their personal responsibility for their own healing and health.

Quality of One Level 1: With the Vortex Pendent and the techniques taught in this seminar, we can once again achieve our natural, vertically oriented energy system. David Wagner has recognized verticality as the basic precondition for consciously experiencing unity with All That Is. The main focus for Level 1 is the conversion to verticality and the associated purification of the entire energy system.

Quality of One Level 2: The second level of the Quality of One process leads to an expansion of the now stable, vertical energy system and to an increase in the amount, quality, and speed of energy that can flow through it. The imparted techniques show ways of sharing this expanded potential with other people and actively participating in the healing and development of the entire planet.

Tachyon Practitioner Training Level 2: The combination of the application concepts taught in the Practitioner Training Level 1 with the capabilities achieved in the Quality of One Level 2 seminar opens up unique treatment paths that previously did not exist. The use of organ-specific tachyon products, which transform the entire organs and organ systems into tachyon antennas, is currently limited to the successful graduates of this training.

As a foundation working on a non-profit basis within the scope of the worldwide active peace organization "Peace 21," the **Tachyon Institute** will support the trainers, course participants, and other people who are interested. Free and independent, it will be dedicated solely to working for the peace of the individual and all of humanity.

The future has begun! We now have the aids for gracefully developing into the humanity that the Creation intended us to be. I invite each of you to lay aside the powerlessness, fear, and ignorance regarding the consequences of hundreds of years of power abuse, exploitation, and blindness toward nature; to resolve past and present personal entanglements and risk a quantum leap in your own healing and development, and into the awakening of your true nature! This is the mightiest gift that we can give ourselves, Mother Earth, and life itself.

May peace prevail on earth!

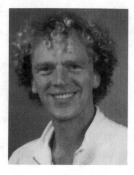

About the Author Andreas Jell

Born in 1958. Trained in chiropractic, naturopathy, acupuncture, and psychotherapy. As a leader in Tantra groups and shamanistic healing work, he strives for holistic healing and development. Only since he has begun using David Wagner's Tachyon technology has he felt that this objective is being achieved with 100% accuracy. This current book is meant to equally encourage patients ("sufferers"), therapists ("healers"), and truth-seekers to risk the quantum leap into the new consciousness of healing and development. This new consciousness can simultaneously do justice to the most modern findings of physics and the most ancient mystic, spiritual experiences—marrying science and spirituality into a new paradigm of medicine and spirituality. Together with this new consciousness, the use of Tachyon energy will represent the medicine of the next millennium.

Author Andreas Jell has been trained by David Wagner, the inventor of the Tachyonization process, as a teacher for the Quality of One Seminars and a trainer for the Tachyon Practitioner Training . Within the scope of the Tachyon International Institute for Spirituality and Technology, he dedicates himself throughout the world to training highly qualified trainers and propagating a lifestyle that expresses love, peace, and respect for oneself, fellow human beings, and the entire Creation.

Sources of Supply
www.tachyon-energy.com

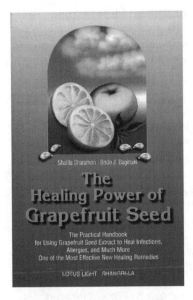

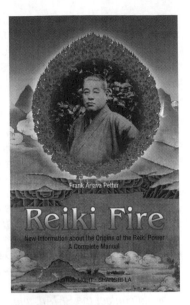

Shalila Sharamon · Bodo J. Baginski

The Healing Power of Grapefruit Seed

The Practical Handbook for Using Grapefruit Seed Extract to Heal Infections, Allergies, and Much More. One of the Most Effective New Healing Remedies

Latest scientific studies show that plant extract from grapefruit seeds has a large range of effects and applications for both internal and external use in preventative health care, therapy, cosmetics, and baby care. Based on international research, two bestselling authors have compiled sensational therapy successes and areas of application for this biological broad-spectrum therapeutic agent, antibiotic, antimycotic and antiparasitic, preservative, and hygienic agent of the future. In addition to scientific proof, this practice-oriented book includes proper dosages and procedures.

160 pages · $12.95
ISBN 0-914955-27-6

Frank Arjava Petter

Reiki Fire

New Information about the Origins of the Reiki Power A Complete Manual

The origin of Reiki has come to be surrounded by many stories and myths. The author, an independent Reiki Master practicing in Japan, immerses it in a new light as he traces Usui-san's path back through time with openness and devotion. He meets Usui's descendants and climbs the holy mountain of his enlightenment. Reiki, shaped by Shintoism, is a Buddhist expression of Qigong, whereby Qigong depicts the teaching of life energy in its original sense. An excellent textbook, fresh and rousing in its spiritual perspective, this is an absolutely practical Reiki guide. The heart, the body, the mind, and the esoteric background, are all covered here.

144 pages · $12.95
ISBN 0-914955-50-0

Herbs and other natural health products and information are often available at natural food stores or metaphysical bookstores. If you cannot find what you need locally, you can contact one of the following sources of supply.

Sources of Supply:

The following companies have an extensive selection of useful products and a long track-record of fulfillment. They have natural body care, aromatherapy, flower essences, crystals and tumbled stones, homeopathy, herbal products, vitamins and supplements, videos, books, audio tapes, candles, incense and bulk herbs, teas, massage tools and products and numerous alternative health items across a wide range of categories.

WHOLESALE:

Wholesale suppliers sell to stores and practitioners, not to individual consumers buying for their own personal use. Individual consumers should contact the RETAIL supplier listed below. Wholesale accounts should contact with business name, resale number or practitioner license in order to obtain a wholesale catalog and set up an account.

Lotus Light Enterprises, Inc.

P. O. Box 1008
Silver Lake, WI 531 70 USA
262 889 8501 (phone)
262 889 8591 (fax)
800 548 3824 (toll free order line)

RETAIL:

Retail suppliers provide products by mail order direct to consumers for their personal use. Stores or practitioners should contact the wholesale supplier listed above.

Internatural

33719 116th Street
Twin Lakes, WI 53181 USA
800 643 4221 (toll free order line)
262 889 8581 office phone
WEB SITE: www.internatural.com

Web site includes an extensive annotated catalog of more than 7000 products that can be ordered "on line" for your convenience 24 hours a day, 7 days a week.